SO YOU WANT TO BE A VET?

The Realities of Studying and Working in Veterinary Medicine

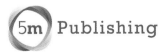

Publishing

SO YOU WANT TO BE A VET?

The Realities of Studying and Working in Veterinary Medicine

NEIL PATON

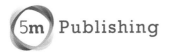

First published 2015

Reprinted 2016, 2018, 2019

Copyright © Neil Paton 2015

Published by
5M Publishing Ltd,
Benchmark House,
8 Smithy Wood Drive,
Sheffield, S35 1QN, UK
Tel: +44 (0) 1234 81 81 80
www.5mpublishing.com

A catalogue record for this book is available from the British Library

ISBN 978-1-910455-08-1

Book layout by
Keystroke, Station Road, Codsall, Wolverhampton

Printed by
Bell & Bain Ltd, Glasgow

Photos by Neil Paton

With thanks to my wife Celine for the patience while I wrote this, and my children Juliette, Charles and Nicole for the smiles between writing sessions!

TABLE OF CONTENTS

1
INTRODUCTION

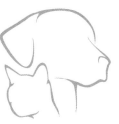

WHY HAVE I WRITTEN THIS BOOK?

In the summer of 2012 a letter that I wrote appeared in the *Veterinary Times* replying to a colleague who believed that undergraduates were unprepared for veterinary practice as these bright, motivated and idealistic students were broken by the university system and the profession as a whole. My response defended the profession and its members, as they are a diverse, hard-working and caring bunch. I offered to teach any potential applicants that my fellow contributor felt were unprepared on a course that I run with colleagues at an agricultural college in South Wales. This course focuses on farm animals and this book is an extension of the aims of that course.

This course was developed after a discussion over coffee one day where the subject was how school pupils could get experience for applications to veterinary school. The result of that conversation was a week-long course on farm animal veterinary medicine for potential applicants. The planning of that course and the thoughts that have gone into this book are the same.

Preparation is a large part of the success of anything. A career in veterinary medicine is no different. Part of the preparation is determining whether the career is right for you. This book is part of that and an attempt to give potential applicants an insight so that only those most suited to the profession will apply. There may be misconceptions about the career among applicants and those that are supporting them in the application process, through education and their career. Through this book I am hoping to correct these misconceptions so that the decision – and the support to make the decision – is based on the correct perception as much as possible. This preparation will hopefully contribute to a reduction in the mental health issues that concern the profession currently. Not only have I known colleagues of mine from school and early college training that have committed suicide, but there is a high level of mental health issues within the profession and many members use alcohol to cope with the demands of the career. Veterinary surgeons work long hours and may work in areas or practices that have little support professionally or clinically. This can be as a result of the remote location or the culture of the practice that graduating veterinary surgeons find themselves working in. This can be a contrast from the university course where there are trained and experienced staff to provide support. Fellow students who are going through the same stage will also be there to provide emotional support.

The long hours put physical pressure and mental stress on the individual veterinary surgeon. The work that is carried out can be of two contrasting types. First, it can be mentally challenging and this can increase the mental exhaustion of the veterinary surgeons, as it may have to be done when the full picture is not known and important details have to be hazarded at. The other type of work is of a routine and repetitive nature, where there is little opportunity for intellectual challenge, such as testing cattle for tuberculosis or vaccination of animals. The tasks are relatively easy to learn but the level of attention must remain high in order to pick up on those animals that do require further investigation and may require further work. Both of these will induce frustrations in veterinary surgeons that may lead to mental stress and illness. If this goes wrong then the client may complain and without balancing praise, it can appear that the feedback is all negative, which will add to the potential for illness. The curriculum trains students to be self-critical and this can compound feelings of failure.

All of this is done in an environment that requires hard physical effort that will sap the reserves of the veterinary surgeon.

The contrast between the support in university and that frequently experienced in practice is huge. The transition from a course where intellectual challenges are almost daily to a job where routine and repetition are more normal is not an easy one to make.

Veterinary surgeons are a highly motivated bunch and extremely self-reliant, and the people involved in the profession can be highly competitive. On the surface this is a good set of attributes to have, but they can be counterproductive. Once a problem has started then it can be difficult for many to seek help, whether that is from colleagues or professional organisations. So attributes such as being empathic but not emotionally involved, being self-critical and highly self-sufficient may all predispose the veterinary surgeon to mental illness. This can manifest as alcoholism, depression and suicide.

All of this was circulating in my head when the discussions about developing the course were being held over many cups of coffee. Our thoughts were that we needed to prepare students as best we could for the realities of farm animal veterinary practice realities. Like that course, this book is an attempt to let prospective students get an accurate idea about what veterinary surgeons get up to on a day-to-day basis, so that anyone reading this book can have enough information in order to make a rational decision about joining the veterinary profession. Part of producing a successful student on any course is ensuring that the correct students are recruited to the course, and this book and the course are an attempt to help that process.

WHO AM I?

I am a lecturer and I teach veterinary students in their clinical years. This is stimulating work, as the students present frequent fresh views and enthusiasm, but my career has taken in a lot of other types of veterinary practice. As a young Scot, I started as most students do, working at my local veterinary practice in Angus and after a gap year teaching English to Tibetan refugees and harvesting on South Uist, I started at the Royal (Dick) School of Veterinary Studies, completing a BSc in veterinary pathology and a Bachelor's in veterinary medicine and surgery. Mixed practice in Aberdeenshire beckoned immediately after graduation, and my beginner mistakes were made there. I was a mixed-practice veterinary surgeon for three years and gained experience with all species, including native wildlife.

A PhD beckoned after that and I conducted basic research on cattle, organising experiments to determine host responses to infection by a food poisoning bacterium. In the period that followed, I worked in overnight emergency practices, farm animal practice and sole charge companion animal practices both in the UK and Australia.

As an undergraduate I took the opportunity to work as a research assistant in the Indonesian tropical rainforest, to conduct pharmaceutical research in the deserts of Jordan and to maintain and improve the health of zoo animals in Thailand.

All of this has led me to my current position of lecturing and living in the south of Wales with my wife and three children on a smallholding raising sheep and pigs. Within Wales I am involved in representing the profession as president of the Welsh branch of the British Veterinary Association and work with the farming industry to eradicate disease.

This is not a boast in order to suggest that I have been everywhere and done everything, but rather to demonstrate that I have a reasonable background on which to base my discussions and interpretations of veterinary medicine as a whole. In some ways, I am not the right person to write this advice. The typical veterinary surgeon of the future will not be a middle-aged male, so it might be more appropriate for a woman to write the book as the profession will be predominantly female in the future. However, I hope I have the empathy to represent our profession in all our various guises.

WHAT DO WE CALL OURSELVES?

I am a veterinary surgeon and that's how I generally describe myself on forms and when introducing myself to others. The job comes with other titles that others who fill the same function in society use – some use 'vet' or 'veterinarian'. These titles are protected and only used by those qualified from an accredited degree course. Upon qualifying as a veterinary surgeon then, as a courtesy, Australia, the USA and most of Europe will allow the use of 'doctor'. In the United Kingdom this has just been allowed in 2015. I intend to use the term 'veterinary surgeon' throughout the book.

A BRIEF HISTORY OF THE PROFESSION

Animals and man have had a long association and it is likely that local healers throughout the ages have tried to treat animals. To this day, the use of ethnic treatments still occurs where the availability of antibiotics and other medical products are unavailable. The first evidence of a named person who was considered as an authority on treating animals occurred around 3000 BC. Called Urlugaledinna, he lived in Sumer in Mesopotamia and worked as a royal physician. There are also documented laws relating to treating animals within the Sumerian Empire. Healing appears to have been monopolised by priests throughout early veterinary history, with the training slowly becoming more formalised with the passing of time, until it became linked with human medicine. Veterinary medicine was developed in the Roman, Greek and Arabic Empires. In the Middle Ages up to the beginning of the Enlightenment, the treatment of animals was carried out by farriers (horses) or cow leeches (farm livestock). In the UK, the Odiham Agricultural Society was instrumental in pushing for animal health specialists and was among the first to push for formal veterinary education. Claude Bourgelat was a Frenchman who was well respected as an expert in horses and their care, and he set up the first veterinary school of the modern era in Lyon in 1762. Between 1762 and 1800 there were 19 veterinary schools opened in Europe. One of these was the London Veterinary School in 1791, the first veterinary school opened in the United Kingdom. A graduate of Lyon, Vial de St Bel, was the first professor of the London Veterinary School, which later became the Royal Veterinary College. Iowa State University is the oldest state veterinary school in the United States. Older private courses were established but are now defunct. A graduate of Edinburgh founded Ontario Veterinary College in 1862, making that Canada's oldest veterinary course. Melbourne Veterinary School is the oldest in Australia.

The methods used have paralleled those in use in human medicine, with disease first being ascribed to spirits, and prayers and rituals invoked to rid the animals of disease. Humours have been blamed, with bloodletting being used to 'balance' these. Surgical techniques involved lancing abscesses or bloodletting for thousands of years. Firing was later used to increase healing as the teachings of Hippocrates and Aristotle gained influence on medicine. It wasn't until the Enlightenment that this started to change.

WHAT I INTEND TO ACHIEVE

The veterinary profession has a long history but the true popularity came with the books that were written by James Alfred Wight – using the pen-name of James Herriot, a veterinary surgeon in Yorkshire. These books are really easy to read and paint a picture of the job that is romantic and satisfying. The popularity and romance of the books and the later TV series saw an increase in the number of applicants to university courses due to the increased attention paid to the profession. I have read a few of the books and I must stress that they are not representative of the veterinary profession as members today experience it. As with the course, it is my intention with this book to try and give readers an accurate picture of what veterinary surgeons are involved in when they get up and go to work.

So this book provides an overview of the veterinary profession and will help you to understand the profession as it is and as it might be. It will hopefully make you think a little harder about the issues that the veterinary surgeons face on a day-to-day basis. It will also consider the range of careers that you can undertake once you qualify from the university course. Being a clinical veterinary surgeon like James Herriot is only one of the options available.

Over the course of the book I will discuss the requirements for getting into veterinary university courses, but I hope to convince you that these requirements are not just hurdles you have to jump but have a deeper function in helping you decide your career. The course will be outlined to allow you as a prospective student to get a flavour of what you will be getting involved in.

Veterinary medicine is a small but important part of working with animals, so how we fit in as part of a team is important, as are the issues that the profession currently faces and will face in the future. All of this will be discussed and will hopefully allow you to think about areas of veterinary medicine and the profession that you may not have considered before.

The final career that you decide upon will depend on your interests, and this book will consider the full range of careers available to you. It will look at some of the things going on in veterinary clinics and farms. Veterinary surgeons also contribute to science, politics and the development of countries that are still developing, and we will consider what has been achieved in these areas. These issues all have ethical and welfare implications, and these will be discussed by looking at how veterinary surgeons have dealt with them and what still needs to be dealt with.

Veterinary surgeons love acronyms and we will look at a selection of these to explain what they are and to give further insight. These will mainly be the organisations that are involved in veterinary medicine.

The economics of veterinary medicine will be looked at, from the costs of courses that students will have to pay, through to national disease problems. The salary that a graduate can expect to receive throughout their career and the value of veterinary treatment will be looked at, and in both cases the perception of the public of high salary and expensive treatments can be considered.

The profession is a fast moving one with changes happening all the time, it is very difficult to predict what changes will happen but I will have a go at future gazing.

WHAT IS NOT INTENDED

This is not a textbook of the veterinary profession and veterinary medicine. It is intended to provide guidance to areas that I felt might be of interest to the reader. The subjects are not covered comprehensively as that would be a veterinary curriculum in its own right. I have simplified some things, hopefully not too much and not in a misleading way but further reading might be helpful in areas where interest is piqued. Some interesting websites are included as references.

My hope for this book is that you – and whoever you discuss your options with – use it to help make a good decision. That decision may be to join the profession or not. The decision is yours but I hope that this book helps.

2
BECOMING A VET

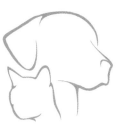

> ## KEY POINTS
>
> - Work experience should help you to decide whether being a veterinary surgeon is the right choice for you.
>
> - The academic requirements are very high and places are limited.
>
> - Some courses will require additional examinations – the biomedical aptitude test (BMAT).
>
> - The courses all cover the same areas but the approach to teaching will be different and you need to be comfortable with the way of teaching.
>
> - The course is a five-year commitment.
>
> - Outside activities are very important for many reasons – even at university a balance between work and play must be struck.
>
> - There is a requirement to attend veterinary practices through the holidays, which means that the ability to work summer jobs is limited and may mean more loans are needed.

The first part of any journey in the veterinary world is training, whether that is at the advanced stage of carrying out sophisticated and pioneering surgery or being the face of veterinary politics, but everyone has to start somewhere and for most vets the training and preparation starts well before the first day at vet school. If you choose this course then you will be learning and training for the rest of your life! As in most things, we should start at the beginning of a vet's career and get that right before moving onto more complicated things.

Most veterinary students decide that they wanted to be a vet at a young age and hold on to this desire throughout their school career, sacrificing many weekends off and social activities along the way. Such commitment is necessary; as you are no doubt aware, the entrance to get into veterinary school is highly competitive. In common with a number of other careers, a degree of work experience is required and expected before you enter the course of study, as well as the academic requirements of the institution. In the UK, most careers guidance staff and teachers who give advice on possible career paths will suggest that a student tries to spend weekends with a vet and see what the career involves. Certainly this is how I got my first taste of the career in Scotland some 20 years ago.

YOUR FIRST EXPERIENCE WITH A VET

Even at this early stage of your budding career there are certain expectations if you are to get the best out of your time at any vet practice. These are important because it's not just the time that you spend at the vet's that is important, but the depth of experience that you get within that time. This approach will stand you well in your career and studies. We will come to that as we go on, but why are there such expectations on you from day one? There are a number of reasons: first, the veterinary profession deals with the public each day and you will be at least part of the image presented by the vet; second, the veterinary environment is frequently a busy place and the staff are working very hard, which should be respected; finally – and especially where large animals are involved – the vet is responsible for the safety of everyone in these environments so you should, as far as possible, be vigilant for possible dangers.

As you are likely to be meeting the public as part of your time at the practice, you should do the vet the courtesy of matching their level of dress. It's probably wise to discuss this with the practice before you go, but neat and professional should be the aim. Suitable clothing for the type of work planned is always sensible. If you are likely to see practice with a farm vet, then you are likely to get wet and it's important not to spread diseases, so something that can be easily cleaned after visits is required. If you have taken this into account, then the vet is probably going to enjoy engaging with you and you will therefore get more out of your time.

All animals are potentially able to cause harm and you should use your time to learn how they react so that you can anticipate an animal's reaction in the future. Remember vets deal with animals that are in pain, scared and distressed. It's important not to get in the way, as you may get hurt and you may compromise the animal's care. This is an important educational experience – so never be afraid to ask where you should stand or let the vet know if you are unsure about being near the animal.

Enthusiasm and politeness are important and you will get more from the majority of vets if you are willing to get involved but remember your limitations.

What should you expect to get out of this early experience of time spent with a vet? 'The more you put in, the more you get out' is a typical statement for this type of experience but that doesn't mean that it's not true. The more enthusiasm and interest you show, the more involved the vet will become with you. I don't mean that you should expect to be involved in surgery, but if you are keen and help out in return for the time invested in you – for example, make the tea, sweep floors, clean cages – then most vets are likely to go the extra mile and discuss cases and concepts with you.

Students at all stages will often try to get as varied an experience as possible. A word of warning, however: there has to be some depth to the experience. To get the full depth of experience that is available means that you have to put in the time with each practice – staying with one practice for a good length of time will allow you as an observer to follow cases from beginning to end.

In all cases, what does the university system look for in the experiences that you have achieved in your time with the vets? They don't expect you to understand all the details of each case, but will require evidence that you have been thinking about the various aspects of each case. This could include the ethical and welfare aspects, the use of diagnostics, the economic issues associated with the case you have seen or the political dimensions of current issues that may have been raised by your experience.

LOOKING AFTER ANIMALS

A good part of your studies will look at how animals are kept, how they are fed and what uses we put them to. This may be as pets, wildlife or as animals that feed us in many ways – from milk to meat – and clothe us with leather or wool, not all of which is from sheep. Other uses include medical and scientific research to improve our understanding of the way the world works.

A lot of vet work involves helping the keepers of the animals to maintain the health of the animals for which they have responsibility. Within the course (which we will talk about later in much more detail) a large emphasis is placed on understanding how to keep animals and you should probably start learning about these as soon as possible.

It's important to become comfortable with animals and getting a basic understanding of how they will react when placed in various situations. Ensuring you are in the correct place to observe and are not in the way, or being competent to handle the animals will improve your work experience before university and throughout the university career.

The next point to make is that looking after your own pet is as important in this respect as going to a zoo on the other side of the world (although if you have the chance to do this – go!) but if you can't get these opportunities, remember that it's better to have some depth to the time looking after animals than a quick visit with no involvement. If you have a specific vet school in mind, it's wise to look at its requirements for work experience.

Looking after animals – whether it's being a vet or milking cows – tends to involve long hours and hard work. It also can be frequently unpleasant (I still get cold and wet on visits to farms, and lunch can be a long time coming), with long days and cold conditions. It's important that you are prepared for this. If you find that it's not for you then it's not a cause for embarrassment – there are careers I would not be able to cope with. One of the reasons I am writing this book is to ensure that those who are interested in being vets are as fully prepared as they can be. I organise the course mentioned in the first chapter to allow people get experience on a farm as an insight into the agricultural industry. The delegates that attend that course are assured that if, at the end of the course, they decide that they will not go on to train as vets, the course organisers and I will still regard our task as successful as long as they are clear about the reasons for their choice. In your work experience, you should aim for a similar level of knowledge.

WORK EXPERIENCE REQUIREMENTS

There are no veterinary schools that will accept an application that has no evidence of experience with animals. It is important to check with your favoured veterinary course what the requirements are. This can be done by contacting the university directly, checking its website or looking in the prospectus.

The quality of experience is as important as the duration, although it is difficult to get quality without sufficient time. This time should be used to get a basic understanding of how animals are kept and used, preferably in a professional setting. This can be on a farm, at a riding stable or in a pet shop. It is important that you question everything that you see and try and understand why things are done and be able to explain and, better still, critique what you see. This extends to the time spent observing a veterinary surgeon when deciding whether you want to be a vet or not.

GETTING WORK EXPERIENCE AT A VETERINARY PRACTICE

As the veterinary profession is so competitive, it can be difficult to get work experience places at a particular practice. Other prospective veterinary students will be trying to get places and those already on the course will be taking places as well. There are not an infinite number of places available and careful planning will be required if you are to get into the practice you want. Being flexible with the dates that you can attend will help, as the practice can offer more options to you.

Work experience with a veterinary surgeon that fulfils your needs may mean asking for time with a veterinary surgeon that deals with an area of the veterinary business that your local practice doesn't deal with. This can be difficult, but the Royal College of Veterinary Surgeons (RCVS) has a website that can help you find a veterinary surgeon who deals with that aspect (http://findavet.rcvs.org.uk/find-a-vet), whether that is exotic animal species, farm animal health or public health. The Australian Veterinary Association has a similar section on its website for work experience (www. ava.com.au/findavet) as does the New Zealand Veterinary Association (www.nzva.org.nz/find-a-vet). There is no equivalent website in the USA, so you may have to resort to the phone directory or using the internet (both of which are options in all parts of the world!).

Contact the veterinary practice in plenty of time; be clear about what you want and what stage you are at in your plan to become a veterinary surgeon. Consider telling them what you would like to get out of the time at their practice. This will allow them to attempt to match your expectations and their work, even if this means letting you know that what you expect is too advanced or not what they actually do on a day-to-day basis.

IT'S NOT ALL ABOUT ANIMALS!

When discussing the application process, we should consider the other things that veterinary schools are looking for!

I was talking to an old lecturer of mine (one that I worked well with and also did holiday-time projects with), and his take was that we should look for colleagues that will add to the life of both the college that they are joining and, ultimately, the profession that they are joining. Incidentally, the scariest lecturer I knew was of the opinion that we should all read an entire newspaper daily in order to keep us interested in the world about us. Although they had very different attitudes to the students studying at their institution, the messages of these two lecturers are the same – you are not expected to be solely interested in animals to the exclusion of all else. Colleagues of mine have been martial artists, rugby players, professional football players, musicians and climbers. In the profession we have authors of historical novels and runners who compete at the national level. Looking at sites for American universities, they also look for involvement in the community and leadership activities. Here again, universities are looking for evidence that you are going to add to the community in which you live and work, both as a student and a qualified professional.

MAKING A DECISION

There is a more serious note to this process, which I think summarises why applying to a veterinary course should be approached as more than just a tick-box exercise. These requirements should not be merely viewed as hoops through which you have to jump to get into the school of your choice. The veterinary profession has a problem that expresses itself in a worryingly high suicide rate. There are complex reasons for this and it is neither my desire nor possible to cover all the reasons here. I will just reiterate the point that I have tried to push in this section, that you should take the chance before you apply to understand as much as possible about the career you are about to start.

Don't be too downbeat though – it's a great career and I would encourage you to become a vet but it has to be *your* decision – not one that is made by your parents, friends or teachers.

ACADEMIC REQUIREMENTS

There are many myths about being a vet and we will mention them as we get to the appropriate points. One thing that is not a myth is that you need to get good grades to get into veterinary school. The specific academic grades are variable between countries and schools, but it is unlikely that anything but the best grades will be accepted – whether that is A*–B grades, 30+ points or some other grading notation, such as a high grade point average as is used as part of the evaluation in the USA.

The academic grades will also need to be from the sciences, as veterinary medicine is at its heart a scientific subject. A strong grounding in maths and particularly statistics is helpful, as much of the evidence-based medical thinking is based on statistics. Assuming that the intent is to study and work in a country where the main language is English then a strong grounding in this language will help; communication (oral and written) is a critical skill in all of the aspects of veterinary medicine. If the ambition is to work or study in countries where the main language is not English, then a good ability with the appropriate language will be required.

The grade requirements will shift from year to year and from university to university so it would be impossible to list them in any sensible format; each favoured university should be checked individually.

The universities will also want to check your aptitude for the course. Asking prospective applicants to sit the biomedical aptitude test (BMAT) does this. This test is a written exam that typically takes two hours to complete. Through three sections it tries to show that the applicant has an ability to think logically through problems, analyse data and communicate ideas effectively and clearly. Not all courses require this test, but it does form part of the requirements for many.

One implication of this requirement for excellence in academic achievement is that all of the new applicants will have this high standard. This can be a difficult transition for the unprepared, going from being the highest achiever in a school to one of many attending the veterinary course. It may require an adjustment of expectations about what is achievable and what success will look like.

APPLICATION

Application to a veterinary course in the United Kingdom is through the UCAS system. This manages the applications to all the courses from all the applicants in the UK university system. If a course is not filled then a process called 'clearing' is used to match students that have not gotten a preferred place to a place on another course. The popularity of the veterinary medicine courses is such that no places will be unfilled and clearing is not an option for an applicant.

In the United States there is a similar system – the Veterinary Medicine College Application Service (VMCAS) – that all students must use. This system can allow application to both veterinary courses in the USA and in New Zealand, and is required for US students applying to some colleges abroad. In some cases direct applications will be accepted.

The application process is a stressful time and it would be sensible to ensure that enough time is given so submission deadlines for all the required documentation are not missed.

THE VETERINARY COURSE

A common myth is that veterinary surgeons train for seven years – longer than a doctor! You may be relieved to hear that this is not true. Undergraduate courses in both medicine and veterinary medicine are five years long. After graduation, those qualifying in medicine will go into further training, but a veterinary graduate has the option of starting in private practice the day after graduation.

There are as many ways to arrange a veterinary course as there are veterinary schools, and as many ways to teach as there are lecturers in the universities. Some will work for you and others may not. Therefore it's important to be aware of these differences and then decide which type of course suits you.

Some schools use a spiral curriculum and integrate all the aspects of teaching from day one. These courses will frequently revisit body systems at least twice during the full course: initially as a course concentrating on the fundamental sciences associated with the system, then returning to the body system with a clinical context.

Other courses provide a solid science-based foundation (the teaching may be with non-clinical classmates). They will teach biochemistry and physiology, for instance, before going on to deal with clinical teaching in more detail later in the course.

The delivery of information is an important part of your choice, of course. The possibilities are lectures, small group tutorials, electronic means and directed learning.

Even within these categories, some are more designed to signpost where you should be reading and others are more information-dense. Some universities place more emphasis on tutorial groups, while others will emphasise large group teaching.

Within the veterinary course you will study a number of topics (disciplines) either solely or integrated over the whole course. These include anatomy, biochemistry, physiology, pharmacology, ethics and welfare, legislation, pathology, surgery, internal medicine, dermatology, epidemiology, animal husbandry, public health and more.

In the American education system, the veterinary degree is typically taken as a second degree. This allows universities that offer a veterinary course the chance to guide their prospective students through peer mentoring.

Some of these universities have pre-vet associations where veterinary students and those working towards getting onto the course can meet and discuss things like the choice of courses suitable for applying to the course.

In the UK, Australia and New Zealand, as the course is a first degree, there is not the opportunity to provide a similar type of support. Peer support is provided through mentors in the clinical years. This can be quite informal, but increasingly veterinary students who volunteer for this role are given training so that they provide effective help.

DISCIPLINES STUDIED IN VETERINARY SCHOOL

Anatomy

If we are to ask the majority of non-vets what vets know about then I would predict that anatomy would be commonly given as the answer. This is the study of the normal structure of the animal. This encompasses gross anatomy – the skeleton, muscles and organs that can be seen without microscopes or other equipment; it also includes the normal microscopic anatomy (normally referred to as 'histology'), and students will spend a long time looking at and learning to understand the arrangements of cells within all of the tissues.

As you have almost certainly been told, veterinary surgeons are required to understand and know about all animals and this is true but we don't study all the animals individually – the course is quite full enough as it is. Instead we use the common domestic species (dog, cow and horse) as model animals to learn in detail and then use these to understand the differences in other species that we come across either in our studies or professionally. There are a number of reasons why the study of anatomy is required, the surgery teaching will rely and build on the knowledge of anatomy to understand approaches to organs to minimise the chances of iat-rogenic injuries (those caused by the treating professional). Understanding what a normal animal organ or section from tissue looks like is a basic skill in many of the diagnostic disciplines, such as pathology.

The study of this is a very practical subject, with dissection of cadavers being a central part of the training in most, if not all, veterinary school training. It is unlikely that this will change but – as in the modern medical school – training simulations will increasingly complement training using cadavers. A concept that is increasingly important in the veterinary world is 'reduce, refine, replace', which encourages minimal use of animals. It is likely that this will encourage change but it is unlikely that the use of cadavers will be eliminated and it may be inappropriate that veterinary students are not exposed to cadavers.

Biochemistry/molecular biology

This is the study of the processes within cells and the reactions that allow the animal to conduct the functions associated with normal behaviour. This includes understanding the DNA molecules' role in passing on genetic traits to offspring and the role of enzymes in providing nutrients from the gut in feeding the animal. Once again, understanding the normal is central to realising what processes are being affected by disease, trauma, medical and surgical intervention. These can then be researched and mitigated against as appropriate.

Physiology

Biochemistry really concerns itself with the interactions at the single-cell level. Once we get to how tissues interact, we are in the realm of physiology. If you have studied either biochemistry or physiology then you will realise that this is a slightly artificial split of areas of study and is one of the reasons that many medi-cal and veterinary courses are turning to a more combined system for teaching these courses.

Pharmacology

Allied to the previous two disciplines is an understanding of pharmacology. This is the science of how drugs interact with the biochemistry and physiology of the animal to which they are applied. It sometimes strikes students as a fairly dry subject, but in emergency situations it can become necessary to apply this knowledge with speed and under stress.

Ethics and welfare, legislation

How we regard animals and interact with them as food, draught and companions is one of the fundamental aspects of being a vet. Universities will discuss this in detail to train their graduates in these aspects so that they are well-informed and can make up their own minds within a factual framework. This is not to say that there is one answer to all ethical and welfare questions – many ethical and welfare questions have no single clear answer – but providing the appropriate mental tool kit to students will protect the interests of animals in the world. It's a broad and important area and will be explored in detail in Chapter 8. A lot of the legislation is linked to this and will be mentioned at the relevant points throughout this book.

Epidemiology

The way diseases and populations of animals interact is the study of epidemiology; allied to this is the interpretation of diagnostic tests. This is an important part of public health as it is how we identify the risks and patterns in animal diseases and diseases that cross between humans and other species. This discipline uses statistics to better understand the way diseases pass from animal to animal (including people). As vets are involved in protecting important parts of the food industry – from sea fish to abattoirs – a detailed understanding of epidemiology and public health issues is critical.

Animal husbandry

In much of veterinary medicine it is inappropriate care of animals that is at the core of disease. Farm animals are usually thought of as being the recipients of poor care. In the process of writing this book I am reading *Farmageddon* by Philip Lymbery and Isobel Oakeshott, which is concerned with this issue, but exotic species such as reptile, primate and bird species are also held in inappropriate conditions. Part of the role of the vet is to correct these issues, but training keepers in appropriate conditions is just as important, if not more so. There is currently an active debate about which animals are appropriate to keep in captivity (either privately or in a zoo environment). This is obviously linked to welfare and ethics teaching as well as thinking in the professional sphere. This is once again why veterinary schools are moving away from teaching these issues in silos but integrating them across the course.

Pathology

Understanding how the body fails to control disease by either not responding sufficiently, inappropriately or overreacting is the core of pathology, once again it depends on a thorough understanding of the normal subjects. This allows the veterinary surgeon the best chance of placing abnormal findings in the correct context and make appropriate decisions about the treatment of the individual or the population.

Radio-medicine, internal medicine, dermatology, surgery, etc.

The final group of disciplines are used to control, cure and manage diseases. Radiology is used to image problems within the animal where we cannot see them, initially this meant using X-rays but now encompasses ultrasound, MRI and CT scans. Usually these are thought of as a collection of diagnostic techniques, but increasingly there are techniques from treating animals such as scintigraphy, radiation therapy and more that move from the human sphere to the veterinary sphere. Once the disease has been diagnosed, then the other disciplines such as cardiology, internal medicine, surgery, reproductive medicine, urology and neurology are where training is given to correct the diseases.

Research

Vets are involved in research and the training starts in the undergraduate course. In common with other science degrees (chemistry, biology and others), in order to graduate vets are expected to complete a research project on a topic that interests them. This can be a chance to investigate a question that you have a particular interest in. Alternatively, a lecturer at the university may have a project that you wish to pick up on and study in more detail.

PRIZES AND AWARDS

Throughout veterinary school and in postgraduate training there will be many awards on offer. Pharmaceutical companies, animal health charities, the universities and professional bodies all support student learning by awarding outstanding students who achieve high grades or carry out interesting and relevant projects. If you get awarded one of these then it's an excellent achievement. If you don't then there may be an interesting study in the relationship between getting prizes during university and later career success.

OMNI-COMPETENT – OR OMNI-POTENTIAL?

The veterinary curriculum is always in a state of flux as new ideas about the underlying science, how this relates to diagnosis and new techniques and new aspects of husbandry come in to play, while new drugs are constantly being introduced. With all of this comes a huge amount of information. Ideas about how best to teach this are incorporated from many fields and this is integrated with the profession's desires for its new graduates. Added to this are directives from European and world bodies such as EAVE who influence veterinary curricula. What this means is that the student receives a vast amount of knowledge that is hopefully organised in a useful fashion. The traditional view is that the new graduate should be omni-competent but the change in the profession and the huge amount of information required to achieve this is untenable. The curriculum in most universities is aimed at producing veterinarians that are able to handle a defined number of tasks – referred to as 'day one competencies' and that are assessed in the professional development phase of the new vet's career – as well as having the proven skills and desire to continue to learn. These new graduates have hopefully demonstrated omni-potential and will be able to learn new skills and knowledge effectively throughout their career.

ALTERNATIVE ROUTES THROUGH VETERINARY SCHOOL

The overall aim of the courses offered by veterinary schools is to provide students with the ability to undertake the many career alternatives that come under the very broad term 'being a vet'. However, some may wish even at early stage to look at a subject in more detail, such as pathology or biochemistry. This is generally referred to as an 'intercalated degree'. The department of veterinary medicine at Cambridge University has this concept as a core of its curriculum, with all students who study at that college taking a year extra to gain a degree in a topic. Students from Cambridge are encouraged to study an enormous range of subjects in this year. All other universities offer this as an option for their graduates and it could be a brilliant opportunity for study of a subject of interest even beyond the undergraduate research project of the veterinary curriculum.

In some cases there are students who will complete even more advanced studies such as a PhD. This will allow research into a specific area of interest at a much greater level of detail. Before embarking on this career path, the student will have a degree in a relevant subject and the background knowledge that is likely to lead to the successful completion of a veterinary degree and a PhD programme.

OUTSIDE THE VET SCHOOL – EXTRA MURAL STUDIES

Animal husbandry as has been noted is a critical part of the veterinary profession and the best way to learn is to get involved. The RCVS has always been aware of this and part of the qualification criteria at final year is that the vet student will have completed 12 weeks of animal husbandry extra-mural studies. The range of potential placements is mind-boggling, but UK veterinary schools have their own internal regulations about placements that have to be considered. Australian schools have the same requirements, but no other country appears to demand this.

There are currently seven vet schools in the UK and there are as a rough estimate 1,000 students studying in each one. This means that there are 3,000–4,000 veterinary students looking to increase their clinical experience every year. The pressure on veterinary practices is immense, especially those near a vet school. Once again there is a real debate within the veterinary profession about whether the UK system is something that can continue with increasing veterinary student numbers. It would be a shame if this system was to fail, as it is a valuable aspect of the training in the UK and is valued by all the students that attend veterinary schools wherever they come from. It does come with a few drawbacks, including the pressure on places, the inability of students to work through the holiday periods and supplement income and the variability of the learning experience. These are not unique to trainee vets – as many courses require summer placements – but that does not make the drawbacks easier to deal with. The whole extra mural studies (EMS) experience from pre-clinical animal husbandry to the wide variety of poultry, dairy, exotic, zoo and equine clinical EMS available to the motivated student is one of the most valuable experiences in veterinary education.

As with work experience students before getting on a university course, there are expectations on the student if they are going to get the best out of the placement. This means acting at least in a polite manner, but the standards are higher than they were for the earlier experiences. At the moment, the EMS provision is by the goodwill of the providers, whether these are private vets, government vets or otherwise. What obligation does this place on the vet providing it? That is a matter of debate at the moment, but there is once again real discussion about the provision of this very valuable service and the vets providing this service, as many feel an ethical obligation, but too much pressure from students will compromise this.

That said, I hope that this continues, as a vet I was pleased to have a good student that would develop and show promise and as a lecturer I continue to appreciate the changes in students as they explore new concepts and situations. This, however, requires input from the student as much as the vet. This is obvious within the university system but may be less so in practice.

There are differences between the experience before and after joining the course. This depends on how far along you are within the course. If you are looking at the animal husbandry part of EMS (forgive me, this is an obsession) while on the veterinary course then you are trying to learn in detail how animals are kept, so a large amount of the clinical work will be more applicable, but before you are in vet school you are getting a taste for what we do as keepers of animals and for some of the expectations of the profession by the wider community. In the first few years you are building up a bank of knowledge regarding how to look after animals. There will be a balance between the variety of experiences and the depth of these experiences that you achieve.

If there is one piece of career advice that I would give at this point, it would be that you should trade a little variety for more depth.

Depth and variety are also important in the clinical EMS selection. Here you will learn how the knowledge imparted to you on the university course is applied in practice. Additionally you will hopefully be able to put into practice the communication and practical skills that have been imparted to you. You are a proto vet and welfare should be at the forefront of your mind. It will be at the front of the mind of the vet who invests their time in the new generation, if not all vets. This gives you an obligation to be honest and aware of your abilities. An honest appraisal of your limitations and strengths is required, allied with that is an appreciation that the vet you are shadowing has a stressful job, which they have made more difficult by taking the time to mentor you. This means that there will be times where you will have to take a backseat to client expectations and animal welfare. Remember they are human. At this point you are probably feeling vulnerable and/or unsure – and this doesn't change all that much in my experience!

There are recommended EMS outcomes that are expected of your time with vets. These include improving on the animal handling skills that you developed in your previous experience both before the vet school, during animal husbandry EMS and whatever skills you bring from other areas. Allied with this is an intellectual understanding of the implications – both positive and negative – of the systems that are used in farming across the world. It is also now time to start considering the welfare and ethical implications of how we keep animals throughout the world. We will look how the vets who have continued in the career and those who have moved on to other fields have developed their thoughts about this matter.

THERE IS MORE TO LIFE THAN STUDYING!

I hope that by reading to this point you have come to the conclusion that the workload of getting to graduation is high. Both the level of intellectual requirements and the sheer volume are demanding on the student. It may come as a relief that there is a social aspect to being a vet.

A grumpy and near-retirement lecturer of mine suggested that we would not be rounded people or even rounded vets if we did not make time to read the newspaper every day. I have no intention of suggesting that you have to read the newspaper every day but I am in agreement with the concept that part of your time at vet school is about becoming a rounded person. Veterinary medicine, the animals under your care and your clients need a rounded person.

Social events at the colleges

Veterinary schools throughout the world all hold various black-tie events to mark special dates in their calendar. The biggest in any student's college career is the graduation ball that marks their success and is a chance to celebrate the end of a long period of study with colleagues, lecturers and family. Other events are sports club balls and end-of-year balls.

Colleges will also visit each other to compete in sports events and to discuss issues that are of interest to the student population.

Sports

In most universities there is an extensive range of sports clubs available to the interested person. The types of clubs are so varied that it would be futile to list them. If you can't find the activity that you desire, then you can even start your own club. The oldest clubs in the universities in the UK are probably the rugby clubs.

There are as many sports in the university as there are reasons for participating in sports. Students may bring a history of participating in sports and colleagues and students I know have competed at high levels in football, horse-riding, athletics and many more. Others have attained high levels of proficiency in other sports that they would never have considered before going to college, such as martial arts, badminton or scuba diving.

It might seem that there is an expectation that vets will do well in anything that they attempt. Many are good at their profession and their chosen activities outside the profession but many more play sports for other reasons. Many just participate in these activities to relax, to socialise with other people, to maintain fitness or just to escape all the day-to-day pressures.

Other activities

Veterinary surgeons have a wide range of activities and many of these interests are started in college. Students take part in musical performances, write blogs, fish and participate in a bewildering array of other activities. These are taken up or continued throughout university for all of the reasons given above for taking up a sport. These activities will look good on a personal statement but more importantly, the more rounded you are then the more likely you are to be an effective and long-lasting vet. Being totally focused on one task is not the most productive way to live a life. Vets should have the ability to be an integral part of the community if they desire, and the professional aspect of the veterinary surgeon is only part of that.

Alcohol

In common with many other spheres of life, the social life of veterinary surgeons is linked to the consumption of alcohol. The celebratory balls and various societies all have alcohol as part of the get-togethers that occur. There is nothing inherently wrong in this, as alcohol is an accepted social lubricant and part of normal society. But as has been noted in several places, the veterinary profession has an issue with mental health and this can be expressed by the misuse of alcohol. Being aware of this and realising that drinking a lot may not be normal or appropriate goes a long way towards stopping friends, colleagues or even yourself from becoming ill or getting hurt in some way.

SUMMARY

The path to a veterinary career is quite a long one and will require a considerable degree of effort and dedication from the student who wants to go through the course. Because of this level of dedication, this decision must be carefully considered before the application to a course. If this decision is correct for you, then you are more likely to be successful throughout your university time and through the career after you qualify.

The decision to become a veterinary surgeon can be influenced by many experiences and people. In all cases, the prospective student will work with animals and observe at veterinary practices and these should be used to guide their choice. The experience should be approached with an open mind about the possibility of *not* becoming a veterinary surgeon if it is not the right career for you.

The end point of a course is that a graduate will have the abilities to be able to work in any chosen field and with further study become a specialised veterinary surgeon and – it is to be hoped – retain enough knowledge of the species or areas that they don't work in to render first aid if needed. The approach that each university course will take is different, and you should be sure that you will be comfortable with the method of teaching.

The course will be challenging and finding an escape for the build-up of pressures is important; this can be sport, movies or any of a myriad of recreational activities. These are important to promote a rounded person who will be able to contribute to society with more than the career they have chosen.

This is all part of a long-term commitment of five years at university as well as the time preparing for the application. This should not be entered into lightly – but if you do there are a large number of careers that are available to you.

3

VETERINARY SURGEONS TREATING ANIMALS

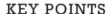

KEY POINTS

- Careful examination and history-taking are key to understanding the disease the animal is suffering from.

- An understanding of the characteristics of the test will aid in interpreting the results.

- Interventions can help but may have problems – both these outcomes must be balanced.

- The emotional impact on veterinary surgeons when euthanasia is carried out cannot be underestimated.

A vet going about their daily tasks has a certain image in the media. The vet is these days dressed in blue scrubs if they are working in a surgery with pets; if they are on farm then waterproof coats and trousers are the more standard uniform; while on equine call, a boiler suit is generally the expected dress. However, with a professional population as diverse as the veterinary one there are many variations and some still stick to a shirt and tie as their professional garb. Whatever the veterinary surgeon is wearing, there are certain things that they all have in common when working with the animal under their care. Vets will collect information from the history and the clinical examination and this will be used to decide what tests might be used in determining the problem and deciding on a course of treatment, whether that requires medicine or surgery.

THE CONSULTATION

There are two parts to the consultation, although these are generally carried out at the same time (vets being constantly under a lot of time pressure). When presented with an animal, the vet will ask questions about the animal – taking the history – and will examine the animal for clues as to the nature of the problem.

History-taking

Taking a good history is frequently crucial to making a diagnosis, will certainly aid in many of the decisions about the animal's treatment and may impact on the treatment of other animals in the household or farm. So what is being asked and why?

- **Age** is frequently asked, particularly of small animals and horses. These animals are more likely to reach an age where problems associated with old age are encountered.

- There are a number of **routine treatments** that are recommended to keep a pet healthy. These include giving the appropriate vaccinations to prevent common and frequently dangerous diseases. Alongside these, giving medicine to control the presence of parasites inside the body, such as worms, and ones outside the body, such as fleas, will control many diseases and will reduce the likelihood of these being the cause of any problem. It may be that you are thinking that this may not be relevant if the dog is lame, for example, but vets also should be looking at the whole management of the animal to anticipate issues that will compromise the animal's wellbeing in the future.

- The **gender** of the animal will influence the range of conditions that the animal will be susceptible to; these may be as obvious as pregnancy – finding out about this may be the point of the examination, so the owner can make sure that the dam (mother) is fed and kept in the best manner possible. Male animals can get diseases associated with the sex glands or may be examined to decide if they can father young.

- **What an animal is fed** can be influential on the disease or the condition; animals can be either underfed or overfed. Underfed animals can struggle to fight off disease or bring up young. In the farm environment, they may not produce as well if underfed or fed inappropriately. Overfed animals may have joint issues as the strain increases with increased weight. Metabolic diseases such as diabetes may be more common or severe in overweight animals.

Breathing difficulties such as coughing, struggling to breathe, and sneezing and nasal discharges are usually signs of the animal having a heart condition. In sport animals, such as racing horses or greyhounds, the signs of heart problems or chest problems may first be noticed as a slowing down or worsening of the ability to exercise.

Vomiting and diarrhoea are frequent reasons for owners of dogs and cats to visit the vet. Careful questioning of the owner may reveal specifics of timing or behaviour that reveal valuable information about the cause. Similarly getting accurate and detailed information about the diarrhoea is crucial to understanding the cause.

Chronic diarrhoea and vomiting can cause significant weight loss, but so can many conditions. Weight loss is, however, an important sign, as it can indicate the length of time a case has been ongoing. Animals that have been ill for a long time can show weight loss and welfare concerns can be raised if an animal is underweight or the history and examination are inconsistent with each other. Equally, weight gain can be an indicator of inappropriate management. In cattle practice, this can indicate issues with feeding or fertility management; sheep can also have related problems. In companion animals, an increase in weight may be an indicator of neglect as overfeeding can be a welfare issue as well. Weight will be measured as part of the examination, changes can be found by asking the owners.

The urinary system is an important system in all animals. If there are substances that need to be removed and are water-soluble then they can be removed through this system. If the control of this is lost or excessive amounts of metabolites are presented at the kidneys then increased volume of urine may be produced. Irritation or infection may be suggested by increased frequency alongside small volumes. Getting useful information does require that the animal be observed sufficiently frequently. Companion animals are usually observed sufficiently, being usually part of the family.

The animal may be presented to the vet as being lame. Within the dairy industry lameness is a big issue and both the veterinary and farming industry are working to reduce the number of lame cows. Horses are commonly lame and dogs also attend the vet as limping. Asking questions about how long the condition has presented for and if it is getting better or worse can help inform the vet about its progression and about whether the animal will get better and, if so, how quickly.

These and many other questions are likely to indicate to the veterinary surgeon a likely cause, but actually examining the animal is generally required to get closer to a diagnosis and is carried out at the same time in most circumstances.

Physical examination

There are probably as many ways to conduct a thorough physical examination as there are vets in practice. Each practitioner probably develops their own unique style but in all cases the key word is thorough. Developing a systematic style from day one in both your ability to question the owner and gather an accurate history and link that to the accurate physical examination of the animal or animals in question are the best tools for a veterinary surgeon.

There are many species that veterinary surgeons are concerned with, but there is a core method to examining all animals. In university I was taught the method that I will outline here, but other methods are equally viable as long as the results are valid at the end.

Farm animal vets tends to spend a lot of time at the rear end of cows and sheep as they're frequently concerned with the reproductive performance of these animals but even farm vets will look at the head to start the clinical examination.

The front of the animal is a logical place to start. In most animals, the first thing moving from front to back is the nostrils (at this point feel free to think of exceptions), so that is where we will start.

The nostrils

These come in all shapes, sizes and colours and are attached to most creatures we are likely to come across. Despite this variety of nostrils, there are common things to look for. In calves typically we are looking for a discharge from the nostrils and the type of discharge may be important in determining the cause and course of action for the animal or groups associated with it. It is normal for a clear watery fluid in small amounts to be present in and around the nose. If the discharge becomes thicker and is combined with a change in colour, then this indicates an infection. This is common to most species and generally indicates a need for treatment.

The mouth

The mouth is generally a little behind the nostrils but I admit it's a close-run thing. Looking in the mouth can be very useful for many reasons – deciding on the age of the animal, assessing the dental hygiene, determining the ability to eat – and may give indications to the presence of important systemic diseases. How much of the mouth can be seen depends on the species being examined. As a rule of thumb, carnivores (cats and dogs typically) allow more of the mouth to be seen due to the anatomy but attitude may limit the actual examination; wild carnivores such as lions may require further intervention to allow an adequate examination.

Within the mouth we have a number of structures to examine: the teeth, the tongue, the lips, and the lining of the mouth. In sheep and cattle, the emergence of adult teeth can be used to tell the age of the animal. The loss of teeth in all species is usually taken to mean that the animal is old, although poor dental care or trauma may lead to tooth loss. Where production or performance animals are concerned, this information may indicate that the animal will not be able to perform the intended task – whether that is producing food or racing – due to an inability to eat enough food to support the energy needs of the animal. Animals that fall into this category may be removed from the farm or enterprise as it is uneconomical to keep them.

In pet animals it's a little more difficult to age the animal, but the hygiene of the mouth may indicate whether the animal is well cared for. If the teeth are covered in tartar or plaque then this may require specific measures to correct or modify the treatment plan.

Touch and vision are important senses in the consultation and examination but the other senses are also required. When examining the mouth, the smell may indicate that there is a more serious disease going on elsewhere in the animal, with the smell in the mouth being the only indication of a problem. If the animal has serious dental problems then this may present as a foul smell. Owners can accept this as normal due to its gradual worsening (dog breath!) or may bring the animal in for an examination as it is becoming unacceptable to them. It may be an incidental finding at a routine health check. Kidney issues may also produce a bad smell on the breath. Some diseases associated with poor nutrition may produce volatile compounds, cattle are frequently found to struggle just after they give birth and this can be indicated by a fruity odour to the breath.

The eyes

Some veterinarians – veterinary ophthalmologists – undergo further study and gain expertise in the area of the eyes and associated structures. All vets will look at the eyes to get information about the animal. Some farm animal diseases are associated with ulcers and discharge and disease may be only within the eye, although there may be a generalised disease. The eye closing may demonstrate pain in the eye and ulcers may be painful and can be an emergency. Looking at the surface and external structures are usually sufficient but occasionally it may require the use of an ophthalmoscope to look at structures deeper in the eye such as the retina or iris. The conjunctiva around the eye may show a change from the normal pink colour, such as red or yellow.

Function is important to eyes and a basic assessment on the animal's ability to see and how well it can see can be done at this point. This may also be a part of a neurological examination.

Ears

Parasites and infections can reside in the ear and so the vet will check in the ears as part of the routine examination, particularly just prior to vaccination. Finding a problem in the early stages before the owner notices can be important, as doing this can limit the consequences of disease by shortening the time period that damage can be done.

Smell again can be important in detecting a problem and may be the reason that an animal, particularly longhaired dogs, may be brought to the veterinary surgery.

Lymph nodes

Swollen lymph nodes are an indication that an animal has a disease process occurring and this is typically an infection but other diseases may cause swelling. There are many throughout the body but those that reside under the jaw (the submandibular lymph nodes) are the easiest to find in most species. Under the corner of the jaw they are usually very small or difficult to feel. If there is an infection then these will swell as they produce cells to fight the infection. Lymph nodes are associated with specific areas and if only some of the lymph nodes are enlarged then it may be a local problem, such as a tooth abscess, but having many lymph nodes indicates a generalised problem. The number of lymph nodes may not indicate how serious a disease is occurring and further information from the history, physical exam or testing will be required in order to decide on this.

The chest

The chest contains the heart and lungs as well as lymph nodes, oesophagus nerves and muscles, all protected by the bones and muscles of the rib cage. This rigid structure protects the organs but also makes it impossible to touch or see the organs within it. To detect problems within the chest, the veterinary surgeon will use a stethoscope. With this the surgeon can hear lung problems such as airspaces opening and closing due to fluid build-up or crackles from membranes rubbing together. The usual explanation given to listen to the heart is to detect murmurs that suggest valves that are not closing properly. Heart problems can also be found by listening to the rate of the heart, with high heart rates suggesting an inability to get blood round the body fast enough. The rhythm can also indicate both problems within the heart and more general problems.

The abdomen

The muscles and skin of the abdomen contain the stomach, intestines, liver, kidneys and bladder, to name the major organs. It is possible to feel some of the organs by carefully pushing into the abdomen, but pain or fear may lead to the muscles being tense, which will prevent the clinician from feeling anything. Even when the animal does allow its abdomen to be felt, it is very difficult to feel anything, although abnormal masses can sometimes be felt.

The limbs

The inability to move properly is a major problem with many animals and is a common reason for the owner to seek advice from a vet. For cattle – and particularly the dairy industry – it may be the most important welfare and economic concern.

In the equine industry, without well-functioning limbs the animal may not race or work as a leisure animal. Pain when moving will reduce the quality of life for many animals as pets.

Feeling down the limb and comparing the left with the right allows us to detect lumps, pain and heat, which will provide clues to the nature of the problem. Watching the animal move will also help in deciding what the problem is and what can be done about it.

THE REPRODUCTIVE ORGANS

The ability to reproduce is a critical reason for many owners to present animals to the vet. Cattle and sheep are required to breed in order to produce meat and milk as well as leather and wool.

In the males, looking at the outside may be sufficient – looking at the penis and deciding if it is normal. The testicles may also be felt for lumps and to consider how free they are to move within the skin; the consistency may also be considered. This is a routine examination in male sheep prior to breeding. Bulls and stallions are also frequently checked in this manner.

In female animals from large species such as cattle and horses, we can examine only the very outer aspects. To fully examine the reproductive organs, vets will frequently feel within the rectum to check the uterus and ovaries. This can be done to confirm pregnancy or to decide whether there is a problem that may explain why the cow or mare is not pregnant. This can only be done in animals of sufficient size and even some cattle and horses will not allow this.

OUTSIDE THE CONSULTING ROOM

What has been done to this point is to look at the individual animal presented to the vet, which has been examined carefully. As well as this, the vet has asked careful questions to find out information about the care of the animal. There is an additional source of information that may guide the management of the case in the future – the environment that the animal lives in. Many diseases are exacerbated by the way that animals are kept. Exotic animal species frequently require specialised care, with many species of reptiles having quite specific require-ments for temperature, humidity and light (both in time under exposure and the UV wavelength). How the animals are housed (in cages, vivaria or plastic boxes), what they are bedded on (the substrate), access to water and presence of other animals are all important considerations. In some cases, the presence of another animal may be stressful or reassuring, depending on the species. There is an ongo-ing discussion about whether some species are suitable for private owners to keep or if they should be only kept in professional facilities due to the complexity and sometimes the size of their housing requirements. The most extreme example of these would probably be non-human primates, which require large areas to roam, as well as complex social groups and environments that meet all their needs for mental and physical health, which may be impossible to meet at a private home.

Exotic animals such as reptiles, amphibians, birds (particularly parrots) and primates are the most likely to have issues that are likely to be associated with inadequate understanding of the requirements for keeping them, while it is farm animals that commonly attract the public's attention for the standard of their care.

Farm animal husbandry standards are important considerations when consider-ing disease management in these production species. Most production animals (cattle, sheep, pigs, fish, poultry) are kept in large groups and this, along with the economic considerations, make husbandry important in maintaining animal health. Calves getting infectious lung disease are probably the classic example of how disease is affected by the way they are kept. Poor ventilation with low airflow and a range of calf ages will predispose the calves in a shed to getting viruses that affect the respiratory system. Dairy cattle present another area where an understanding of cattle keeping is critical – lameness is probably one of the most common conditions encountered in the national dairy herd. The amount of lameness within a herd is probably influenced by the standard of care within the farm. This can be due to routine handling by the herdsman or the housing that the animals are kept in.

Fish are another production species where the environment that the animals are kept in can have a massive impact on their productivity and welfare. In addi-tion, there are parasitic species (sea lice) that can have an impact on the wildlife surrounding the farm. Treatment can also have impacts on the area around the farm. However, careful management can limit the diseases. Whether in saltwater species, such as halibut or salmon, or freshwater species, such as trout or tilapia, the water quality is as critical to the success of the enterprise as where we keep calves and chickens.

DIAGNOSTIC TESTS

Following the history-taking, clinical examination and consideration of the management of the animals, we now have a lot of information that we can use to determine the likely disease that is affecting the animal. Some diseases are quite closely related or can have serious consequences if missed. It is also possible that there is no clear answer after the examination and further information is required to guide the decision on what disease or condition is affecting the animal or may be required to guide the correct course of treatment.

If we are being precise, then the various parts of the clinical examination are in fact diagnostic tests but mostly what we refer to diagnostic tests are from samples removed from the animal that are processed in some way to give a result. These tests can be carried out on blood, urine, faeces, swabs from wounds or other tissues. Some tests will require quite sophisticated equipment, while others can be carried out with simple equipment. Blood samples are a common source of information and, although they are not the comprehensive source of information that some owners believe they are, they can still be very useful. Blood contains many things: water, protein, antibodies, metabolic compounds and waste materials. We can frequently test for these things to determine a range of things, from whether the animal has experienced an infection by a pathogen demonstrated by a rise in antibodies or increase in white blood cells, the state of the internal organs such as kidneys by rise in urea, and whether the animal is dehydrated by looking at the volume of red blood cells in the blood.

Urine samples are easy to acquire from some species and more difficult to get from others. The sample can be used to determine the function of the kidney, detect infection in the urinary tract or problems with systems within the animal including its energy requirements.

Faecal samples can be used to look for parasites or determine how well the animal is digesting its food through looking for the residues. Bacteria can be grown from the faeces to determine the cause of diarrhoea.

Skin scrapes can also determine the presence of parasites as frequent causes of skin problems in all species. Mites are common causes of scratching and irritation in dogs and sheep.

It is commonly thought by owners that most if not all diseases have a bacterial component and a tablet containing an antibiotic will cure all problems. Many diseases are not caused by bacteria but by other factors but where bacteria are involved it is important to ensure that we can treat properly. Ideally the vet would carry out culture and sensitivity on swabs or samples from the site that is of concern, whether that is a wound or, for example, a milk sample from a dairy cow. This test will tell us what species of bacteria is involved – if there is indeed a bacteria involved – and what types of antibiotics are involved.

ANTIBIOTIC RESISTANCE

You will almost certainly be aware that antibiotic resistance is a growing issue across the world with hospitals in the UK finding methicillin-resistant staphylococcus aureus, and extensively resistant tuberculosis a growing problem across the world. Bacteria become resistant after developing mechanisms that allow survival in the presence of antibiotics. Conditions that allow the development of these abilities include too low doses of antibiotics due to underestimating the weight of animals prior to prescribing the drug, or the course being too short as owners stop the course too early. Other causes are more complex and can be from the swapping of genetic elements between bacteria of different species. There is a massive amount of debate about whether the farming industry and by extension the veterinary industry is responsible for this or the use of antibiotics in human healthcare has more impact. I suspect that such use in the agricultural and veterinary industries has had a relatively small impact on the development of resistance worldwide, but it is not my intention to settle that argument here. What does need to be emphasised is that, as people with the privilege of prescribing antibiotics, vets need to be seen to be prescribing responsibly. This means only using when required, using the correct drug for the correct reasons and for the correct length of time and backing that up with appropriate testing. Monitoring of the outcomes (success and failure) can be useful and problems should be reported to allow the monitoring of potential resistance.

Responsible prescribing of antibiotics would seem to imply that culture and sensitivity testing should be carried out prior to giving out antibiotics – but time is frequently an issue, with animals possibly becoming worse before there are test results to work with. Experience and training combined with good clinical records will allow the selection of a suitable drug. This can be discontinued if the response is not as expected or results are available showing a better therapy.

Antibiotic resistance is a real problem that you will encounter as a vet and being aware of it will allow you to deal with it as is required to protect the welfare of the animal in front of you as well as the welfare of future animals.

MORE DIAGNOSTIC TESTS

We have discussed a lot of tests and there are many other examples that could be discussed. These tests can be carried out at the animal's side, in the back of the practice or may need to be sent away to laboratories where there may be experience or equipment that is not available at the veterinary practice.

These tests are useful in coming to a conclusion about the disease or problem that affects an animal. However, a positive result – whether that is from an X-ray or a blood test – does not always mean that the animal has the disease that the tests suggest it does. These are frequently referred to as 'false positives'. False negatives are the opposite, when an animal is classified as unaffected when in fact it has the disease or condition. No test is perfect and the parameters that help to measure the accuracy of tests are sensitivity and specificity. These parameters have to be used in conjunction in order to decide how much confidence that we can have in a particular result truly reflects the state of the animal. Sensitivity is a measure of our ability to determine that the animal is positive for a disease or condition and specificity is the ability to determine whether an animal is not affected by the condition being tested for. This has led to mnemonics such as 'spin' (a positive highly specific test suggests the disease is ruled in) and 'snout' (a negative highly sensitive test rules it out) being used in much of medical practice. These are, however, misleading, as both parameters must be combined to reliably assess the result of a test. In addition to these, it is important to consider the prevalence of the disease. This is the number of cases of disease in the population of animals (incidence is the number of *new* cases in the population) over a given time period. Prevalence is combined with sensitivity and specificity to calculate the positive and negative predictive values. These indicate the confidence that the vet interpreting the test has in their interpretation.

There is potentially a huge amount of uncertainty as depending on the diagnostic test being carried out, all the parameters may be unknown or only approximated at. Prevalence in particular can be a difficult figure to find and sometimes the estimate is the best we can do.

In order to determine whether the animal has a disease, the vet has carried out a significant amount of work and has come to a conclusion about the animal's disease, and it is likely that they also have some idea of the severity and therefore the possible outcomes of the case. Once this is done, a treatment plan can be formulated and agreed with the owner. The treatment plan can include giving medication by various routes, it can involve surgical intervention or there may be intervention within the way the animal is kept to remove the underlying issues that allow the disease to develop. Of course all of these may be required to alleviate the conditions and prevent recurrence.

In some cases it may be that that euthanasia is the best option for an animal.

POST-MORTEM EXAMINATION

Finding out what the disease is may require an examination of the animal after it has died – a post-mortem examination. An answer to the question about why the animal died is needed for many reasons. This may be because it will inform the treatment or management of an entire group, in some cases a number of animals may be used, as this can give a better answer as one may be unrepresentative, it may give closure to an individual and it may be required for evidence at court cases or for insurance reasons. This is a skill set that all veterinary students are given during their training but will require honing throughout the career of the individual.

As with the clinical examination and history-taking, probably the most important thing about the post-mortem examination is that it is conducted in a systematic manner. Again, this is largely a matter of training and personal preference. It consists of opening the animal and examining each of the organs in detail. This requires use of the senses, of sight, smell and touch in detecting changes within the organs. Finding these changes will allow either determination of the problem that caused the animal to die or be euthanased or it will allow the choice of tests to further define the problem.

Post-mortem examinations can be carried out in the practice, on the farm or at specialised centres – some vets work full time in these centres. These veterinary pathologists have usually undertaken some form of further training in this area. In the UK, the government-sponsored labs carry out this function; in other countries commercial or university labs may fulfil this purpose in addition to government facilities.

MEDICATION

To cure and manage conditions it is a frequent requirement to administer some form of medication. This medication can be given in a number of ways (routes). These can be an oral medication such as a tablet or liquid; an injection under the skin (subcutaneously), into the muscle (intra-muscularly) or into a vein (intravenously). Some preparations are applied to the skin, eye or mouth. Other routes are available (intra-osseous, intra-arterial) but are generally for more specialised reasons. Inhalation of drugs can be used in some occasions. To choose which of these is the correct choice depends on many factors. The drug in question may only come in one option, removing the choice. Other drugs come in many forms; antibiotics generally come in both tablet and injection forms. How long the drug takes to become effective in the animal's body may be a reason to choose one route or another (the organ being treated may mean that this is not automatically intravenous). The species may also influence the choice of route, as antibiotics given orally may cause problems in some species (rabbits have particular issues with some antibiotics).

Compliance

Owners can have a massive influence on the success of any treatment plan and one part of that is giving the medication. Making it acceptable to the owner is one manner in helping achieve a good resolution. Mostly owners are happy with tablets but injections may be preferred in some cases, liquids may be preferred in other cases and the owners past experience or preconceptions can influence this. In the case of antibiotic resistance, owner compliance can influence the appearance of resistance, as full courses may not be given, leaving some bacteria able to survive and replicate.

Types of medication

There many types of medication available to the vet. These can be antimicrobials, ecto- and endoparasiticides, antiseptics, anaesthetics, painkillers, diuretics, drugs to support heart function, antispasmolytics, anti-emetics, vitamins and vaccines. These can be used to treat the underlying problem by removing the organism infecting the animal (bacteria or parasites) or by alleviating the symptoms associated with the condition, such as pain or cardiac arrhythmia.

Side-effects

All drugs have effects and these can be very powerful and helpful, but the other side is that many drugs can also have side-effects or adverse events. These are effects on the animal that are expected in a few cases or may be totally unexpected. There are no effective drugs that will not cause problems on occasion. However, these are not to be ignored. Adverse events should be reported to the veterinary medicine directorate by using a 'yellow form', which will detail the event and medications that you have given to the animal.

The veterinary medicine directorate licenses all medications and this is based on evidence provided by the manufacturer. If this is insufficient then more evidence may be required of the company; however, some rare effects will not appear until the medication is used on very large numbers of animals. This reporting system will pick these up and allow the prescribing advice to be refined and provide safer medicine usage.

SURGERY

The other common intervention that is associated with veterinary surgeons is to carry out an operation on a specific animal. This requires anaesthesia, skills and a considerable understanding of pharmacological interactions, a good understanding of sterility and how best to maintain it, a clear picture of the anatomy, as well as the ability to use the surgical tools and knot-tying skills. Surgery is rarely done by one person; the team in the practice usually consists of the vet who is carrying out the surgery, another veterinary surgeon may induce anaesthesia and monitor the animal's heartrate and breathing rate. A veterinary nurse in many cases may take this role. Veterinary nurses (or technicians depending on the country) are an integral part of the team and are force multipliers, allowing the team to work efficiently. This means that another set of skills that are required are the soft skills of team leadership.

Aseptic technique

Surgery requires the surgeon to make a wound to the animal in order to diagnose or treat the condition; some surgeries are undertaken to allow a more accurate diagnosis to be found. This wound breaks the natural protective layers (skin) that protect the animal and bacteria can then gain entry, breed and cause infection, which can compromise the wound healing, making healing slower, possibly causing the animal to become quite ill for a period of time, and occasionally causing a serious illness, with the animal dying as a result. To prevent this as much as possible, the surgical team has to be as clean as possible and where possible work in a sterile manner.

To do this instruments are autoclaved – placed in a box that can be filled with steam at high temperature and pressure – for a long period of time to kill any bacteria. This means that the tools that are placed in the animal will not carry bacteria into the body and set up an infection. In addition all of the cloths (surgical drapes), gloves, gowns that the surgeons wear and the suture material used to close the wound or tie off blood vessels are also sterilised, although these may be done using more technical methods such as ethylene oxide sterilisation.

The surgeons will themselves have to be as clean as possible. This will require that the surgeon will be scrubbing their arms with an antiseptic solution such as chlorhexidine or iodine in order to reduce the bacteria on their skin. Gowns and gloves are then put on in a manner that ensures that the surfaces that are going to be near or in contact with the animal remain sterile. Once dressed and ready for the procedure then the surgeon will be unable to touch anything outside a defined surgical field and if they have to move then they will have to do so with this thought in mind.

Sedation, anaesthesia and analgesia

Surgery requires anaesthesia to allow it to occur. Anaesthesia is the set of skills that render an animal unable to respond and, importantly, be unaware of the surgical procedures being carried out. How this is carried out depends on the situation the veterinary surgeons find themselves working in. In a farm environment, applying a local anaesthetic that will numb the nerves at the surgical site may be all that is required. When operating in a practice environment, a systemic anaesthetic that renders the animal unconscious may be required.

Local anaesthetics are frequently used in all branches of practice but are probably the cornerstone of farm animal surgery. They are drugs that are injected into areas and they stop transmission from nerves at the site of injection. They may be injected at a distance from the operation site as a nerve block; or may be placed along the site of the intended wound to control the pain from the incision.

Sedation is sometimes required to conduct this in farm and equine surgery. Sedation is different from anaesthesia in that the animal is relaxed but still potentially aware of what is happening. These are frequently administered by injecting into a vein or into the muscle and have a variable ability to control pain.

In companion animals and equine as well as other specialties (exotic, zoo, avian) the cornerstone is general anaesthetic, although sedation and local anaesthesia are used as well. The most common way to administer the agents that maintain the anaesthetised state is through allowing the animal to breathe the gases. It is possible to achieve the same effect by administering the drugs through the vein. In either case, the animal is, as we have said, rendered totally unaware of any interventions that are carried out.

Is sedation safer than anaesthesia?

Frequently owners will have concerns about animals undergoing anaesthesia as it is thought by many owners to be a higher risk than sedation.

Anaesthetics have limited to no pain control effects. Although the animal will not respond during the operation, it will potentially exhibit discomfort or pain during recovery and this will limit the recovery and is a poor welfare outcome for the animal.

Surgical skills

The ability to suture the wounds together is a skill that is commonly associated with a surgeon working in the operating theatre. Various materials are used from catgut – which is made from animal collagen – to stainless steel. The choice of material is dependent on site, reason for the surgery and surgeon's preference. The material is stitched in patterns and the material chosen may be knotted twice at the end and the beginning (a continuous pattern) or each loop may be knotted individually (an interrupted pattern). There are many patterns that can be chosen and again the choice is dependent on the same factors as for the choice of material. The patterns can take the edges of the wounds and place them side by side (appositional), take the wound edges and turn them upwards (everting), or turn the wound edges inwards (inverting); and within these broad categories there are many distinct patterns that may be used. Other more specialised knotting techniques are also available to close blood vessels or other tubular structures.

There are other skills that are exhibited in surgery, such as making accurate and controlled incisions to expose sites or remove lesions. This will make suturing the wound easier and improve healing.

Medication associated with surgery

Surgery requires associated medication to allow the best outcome. The veterinary surgeon can use painkilling drugs which may be similar to aspirin used in humans, or may be similar to morphine and other opioids. They may use fluid therapy; delivering large volumes of fluids containing dissolved salts and sugars. This will aid in cases of dehydration, with renal and other organ competence and in blood loss. This is delivered by inserting a catheter into a vein. The catheter is a plastic tube that remains open in the vein allowing a constant regular flow of fluid into the animal.

Antibiotics can be used in surgery to help treat the underlying condition or in the case of surgeries where true sterility cannot be achieved due to the conditions that the surgery is carried out in.

IS THE INTERVENTION USEFUL?

Drugs and surgery, therefore, can have a benefit and a cost to the animal or the population as a whole. And the vet is required to answer a question: how many animals will I have to give a medication or other intervention in order to make a difference? This can be measured in a number of ways, such as number required to treat, number required to harm, number needed to vaccinate or absolute risk reduction. When an intervention is undertaken, whether that is using medicines or surgical in nature, then there are a number of outcomes that can be potentially seen: the animal can return to normal (the ideal outcome), it can be a partial recovery (such as relief from pain for arthritic limb conditions), there can be no change to the animal's condition and finally the animal can be harmed by the intervention. Comparing the rates of these events can allow conclusions to be drawn about whether the intervention is worthwhile. To do this requires looking at a number of research papers following construction of a well thought-out question regarding the problem such as 'will amoxicillin (a specific antibiotic) be more effective in treating cystitis (bladder inflammation typically caused by bacterial infection)?' and carefully interpreting the data presented in the research papers. This is the basis of evidence-based veterinary medicine. However, even this will not totally answer the question – it will give a numerical answer. In the case of the number required to treat, it might be expressed as: it will require the vet to treat ten dogs with cystitis to achieve a cure in five; alternatively it might be expressed as if we treat ten dogs with amoxicillin we will cause diarrhoea in one animal. A key skill of the veterinary surgeon is balancing these two (and more calculations), explaining the implications of these in an appropriate manner to the owner so that they can make an informed decision.

ALTERNATIVE THERAPIES

There are whole ranges of therapeutic interventions that are placed under the umbrella term 'alternative medicine'. These are popular with many sections of the population including some members of the British royal family. These include homeopathy, reiki, chiropractic medicine, Bach flower remedies, crystal healing, acupuncture and many others. What these all have in common is that the underlying principles are not based on a recognisable modern understanding of the physiology and pathology of disease.

Homeopathy is the use of extremely diluted medicinal products to treat animals. This is based on a mistaken understanding of the causes of disease from the nineteenth century and developed by Samuel Hahnemann. The prevailing hypothesis about disease involved miasmas (bad air) causing the conditions and Hahnemann observed that certain substances, specifically cinchona against malaria, would produce similar clinical signs. He suggested that administration of these to someone suffering from these clinical signs would be a cure. Due to his beliefs, he decided that very low doses were better than high doses. Provings were and still are used to decide on the use of a particular remedy. These require people to take the remedies and note the effects that they feel and these reports are used to decide the conditions that the remedy will be used to treat. Provings on humans are used to determine the use of remedies on animals despite any physiological differences. This approach to medicine extends to vaccinations that are termed 'nosodes' and are produced in the same way through serial dilution and succession (agitation of the diluted solution at every dilution). The research that supports the use of either homeopathic remedies to treat diseases or nosodes is unsatisfactory and is probably a placebo at best. Natural reversion to health and observer bias account for the successes attributed to this system. Homeopathy is not only used in companion animals, although these are the most common recipients of alternative medicine therapies. Farm animals are also treated with homeopathy, with this form of treatment being especially popular with organic farming associations. Prince Charles is reported to be keen on using homeopathy on his farms.

Acupuncture is based on the stimulation of vital points and was originally used by the Chinese as a medical treatment. Needles are placed at these points in an attempt to relieve the symptoms that are exhibited by the animal. This is in the original form thought to improve the flow of Qi (the life force) through the animal. Research has attempted to link this original understanding to the current understanding of biochemical and physiological pathways. Again, when looking at the evidence for the use of this modality on a number of conditions there appears to be no or very weak evidence for the effectiveness of acupuncture on animals.

Chiropractic medicine is the manipulation of the spine with the aim of treating muscle pain and other issues associated with the muscles and skeleton. Veterinary surgeons who use this will apply a small force along the plane of the affected spinal joint to alleviate the pain in the body. Again the underlying philosophy of chiropractic medicine in the human field is vitalism and veterinary treatments are based on this. In both the human and veterinary fields, the evidence base to support the use of this treatment is relatively poor.

These three are some of the most common alternative therapies, but there are many others available to the concerned pet owner. All these diverse alternative therapies have one thing in common; these therapies are based on a traditional concept of health and disease. Many of these – such as life force and miasmas – have been disproven. The welfare of animals is safeguarded by the Veterinary Surgeons Act that restricts diagnosis and treatment to veterinary surgeons.

Veterinary surgeons who use alternative medicines in their day-to-day practice will sometimes describe themselves as holistic veterinary surgeons. The term 'holistic' is from a Greek root referring to the whole or entire thing and is used to suggest that the veterinary surgeon is treating the animal as a whole, not just clinical signs. This is unfair on the remaining veterinary profession, who will take into account the environment of the animal and try and look at all of the aspects of an animal's case; in reality all good veterinary surgeons are holistic.

These treatment options sit with difficulty in the evidence-based medical profession. Although there are requests for these treatment modes and veterinary surgeons who are willing to supply these services, it is the profession's responsibility as a whole to educate the general public about the best evidence for any treatments to ensure that the owners have the best information to make good choices for the animals they are responsible for.

MANAGEMENT AND ADVICE

Sometimes surgery and medication are insufficient to manage the issue. In farm animal practice, the issue may be feeding, housing or other issues. Exotic animals are also frequently kept in less than ideal conditions and correcting the housing, feeding and lighting conditions may be critical in dealing with the animal's problem. With athletic animals (horses or dogs) then controlled exercise and rest are possibilities in addition to the changes in environment for other species. Companion animals are frequently overweight and working with the owner to correct this will help any other problems.

In addition to advising the owners once a problem has occurred, many vets will work with owners to advise them on how the animals should be kept in order to prevent disease. This may range from teeth-cleaning and vaccination to weight control. Food production animals may have housing changes required to increase ventilation, and changes in grazing or feeding to manage growth or parasite burden.

An important part of the task of a vet is to assist the owner in managing the animal in order to ensure that the management is as good as required in order to allow the animals to thrive.

OUT-OF-HOURS

For clinical veterinary surgeons, an important part of the job is the out-of-hours commitment. Typically routine appointments and calls will be dealt with in normal office hours. A vaccination to a dog or horse will be carried out from 8am to 6pm roughly. Some countries and practices have differing hours but at one point the veterinary surgeons will stop seeing routine calls and go home. Emergencies happen at all hours, however, and this needs to be covered by someone. Historically this would be shared by the veterinary surgeons working in the practice. The amount of time any one particular veterinary surgeon spends dealing with emergencies depends on the number of veterinary surgeons in practice.

Concerns that can be dealt with out of hours would typically be expected to be life-threatening but just as frequently they are much less serious (but of concern to the owner). It can be difficult managing the client's expectation to be seen immediately with the need to remain available for genuinely life-threatening situations. Some clients will try to overpay to be seen overnight for things like vaccinations, but to see them could delay your response to road traffic accidents and similar situations that might cause an animal to die where it could have been saved.

The level of service, hours worked and emotional impact of client demands can have a significant toll on the mental and physical health of veterinary surgeons, so some have asked specialist providers to cover the out-of-hours work. Other practices, typically corporate practices, are trying to provide a 24-hour walk-in service for any type of appointment. The impact of these changes is yet to be seen.

EUTHANASIA

Bringing about the end of an animal's life can be a difficult duty for the veterinary surgeon to carry out, but it is an important duty that happens in all branches of veterinary medicine. As the keepers of animal welfare, it is our responsibility to ensure that all animals are given as comfortable and painless an end to life as possible. The term 'euthanasia' is derived from the Greek words for 'good' and 'death', and the techniques used are those that are most likely to achieve this.

Euthanasia is carried out for many reasons: the welfare of the animal, the economics of the situation, the social situation and legal requirements.

If the vet and the owner have decided that the treatment of the animal is not going to prove beneficial to the animal then there may be a decision made to end the animal's life as the disease or condition may not be controllable any other way. This may be influenced by the owners' beliefs and attitudes as much as the statistical analysis. Frequently owners will have attitudes that mean they are unwilling to start treatment plans as they are perceived as too aggressive for the animal's health. Old age is frequently used as a reason for animals not being treated; whether this is valid and whether the vet can or wishes to persuade the owner that age is not a relevant barrier depends very much on the case under discussion. Leaving an animal with an untreated condition will generally lead to a poor welfare problem (unless it is usually a self-limiting disease) and euthanasia can be a good option.

In addition to the owner being unwilling to put an animal through a course of treatment or surgery as it is perceived as being too intense, the owner may not be able to afford the treatment. The owner's ability to afford a particular course of action is dependent on their particular circumstances, so it is impossible to generalise about what is an expensive treatment. As with human medicine, there is a huge range of treatments available and in some areas a course of antibiotics or painkillers may be too expensive to acquire. In other areas, animals may receive thousands of pounds of treatment as there is more ability to pay and health insurance may be available to support the treatment of animals. The appropriate amount used to treat animals is dependent on the situation – whether that is the owner's specific circumstance or the areas that the vet finds himself practicing. When thinking about economic issues in the developing world, it is also worth remembering that the single house cow may be a huge part of the family income or one of the families' major food sources.

There may be social situations that require euthanasia. The owners' circumstances may change and this may not allow the keeping of a pet animal, or the arrival of a new child or other major change in circumstances may mean that the animal can no longer remain in the home. It may be that it is possible and desirable to rehome the animal, but this is not always possible.

Related to the social aspect of the animal's home life is its safety around the home, horse stables or farm yard. Animals that are dangerous cannot be part of a home life, cannot be used on a riding yard and are unlikely to be useful on a farm. When a dog bites the owner's family then they may choose to euthanase the animal in order to avoid further attacks. In some cases there may be legislation in place that authorises the authorities to euthanase a dog that is considered dangerous. This is generally breed-specific legislation such as the Dangerous Dog Act 1991 in the UK and similar regional legislation in Australia. The appropriateness of the legislation may be debatable but as the law stands, euthanasia is a possible outcome.

Animals are currently used in important research programmes and the use of them will likely allow the development of new knowledge and drugs. The animals used in experiments within these programmes have particular procedures carried out. Some of these may have no impact on the animal, a very few (about 2 per cent) of experiments are likely to have a severe impact on the animal. In these cases the animal will have to be euthanased again in order to protect the welfare of the animal as much as possible.

Euthanasia, when it is carried out, should be painless and with minimal stress. In addition to these, the aesthetic judgement of the owners may influence the choice of technique, as some owners may perceive a particular technique as being unpleasant. In addition, the safety of the owner may be an important consideration.

In companion animals, an overdose of an anaesthetic is the most common method for euthanasia. In order to facilitate the administration of the drug then a catheter may be placed in a vein. Some vets may recommend sedation of the animal in order to make all of this easier. The intravenous route is the most common route by which the drug is delivered but other routes are available such as intraperitoneal or intra-cardiac. These options are predominantly used when the other routes are not available. In very small animals, the vet may use an anaesthetic that is able to be breathed in by the animal. Chambers can be arranged to allow the gas to be piped in and slowly increased until the animal is no longer able to breath.

Larger animals – such as farm animals and horses as well as large zoo animals – have to be euthanased for welfare reasons. These can be euthanased in the same manner as companion animals. An alternative to euthanasia by overdose is for the animal to be shot. This can be done with a rifle, a handgun, or a shotgun; additionally a captive bolt pistol may be used to kill the animal. In the case of the guns (rifle, pistol, shotgun) the round destroys the cerebrum, rendering the animal unable to feel or respond to anything. A penetrating captive bolt gun uses gunpowder in a blank round to push a metal rod at high speed into the animals' brain, destroying the cerebrum and once again rendering the animal unconscious immediately. Non-penetrating bolt pistols (stunners) use a mushroom-shaped tip at the end of the metal rod. The force applied will render the animal unconscious but will require further intervention to kill the animal but, as before, the animal will not be able to feel anything that happens after the bolt gun is used.

The impact of euthanasia on the veterinary surgeon

Euthanasia is a difficult subject for the owner, who may be losing a much-loved companion or a huge investment in time and effort if it is an important breeding animal. This can induce a huge emotional stress in the owner. Veterinary surgeons are not immune to this issue and this is one factor that contributes to the increased suicide rate among the profession. Veterinary surgeons are four times more likely to commit suicide than the general profession.

Euthanasia in animals can be a positive event and give an animal a dignified exit but it is a highly emotional event. The grief experienced by the owner can be felt by the veterinary surgeon. Due to the personality type associated with the career, veterinary surgeons will have a great deal of empathy with the animals. If the case has taken a lot of time and work then the veterinary surgeon will also build up a relationship with the animal and the owners. At the end of the euthanasia, both the parties – owner and vet – will potentially be suffering from the beginnings of grief. The owner will be able to go home and start the normal recovery process, while the veterinary surgeon will almost certainly have to conduct another consultation with another animal. This will interfere with any recovery by the veterinary surgeon.

Euthanasia requires a degree of technical skill and it is hard enough to deal with the emotional issues when all goes well. Even when the technical aspects go well, the communication is not always carried out effectively and understanding by the owner can be poor. A perfectly normal part of the procedure such as gasping after death (agonal breathing due to the death of the brainstem causing firing of nerves and arrhythmic chest movements) can be seen as a problem if not explained. Euthanasia techniques can go wrong, needles can slip out of veins, catheters can become blocked and bullets can miss the target area or not achieve the effect that is required. This can affect the veterinary surgeon's feeling of competence and increase the pressure on the individual. Thus the potential grief felt by the veterinary surgeon will be compounded by a feeling of failure and incompetence (whether this is justified or not) increasing the stress felt by the veterinary surgeon. This – alongside other factors – will contribute to the high levels of mental health disease experienced by members of the profession.

The profession does recognise the strain that these situations put on the veterinary surgeons involved and have put together support organisations such as VetLife or the wellness and peer assistance programs supported by the American Veterinary Medical Association (AVMA).

THE VET AT THE ANIMAL SIDE

The vet in the clinic, on the farm, in the yard or at the equine yard has a complex task discussing with the person responsible for caring for the animal what the signs of disease associated with the animal or group are; link that with the examination and findings from that to produce a plan for further testing, which may include the post-mortem of animals in the same group, and treatment. Along with the owner, this should be evaluated along with the vet's knowledge of the likely success of the treatments along with potential side-effects. The success of the treatment plan will be dependent on many factors including the owner's ability to manage the aftercare. The treatment plan can involve surgery, medication or changing the animal's environment to address the problem. Sometimes the animal cannot be treated for welfare or legal reasons and the vet is required to euthanase the animal humanely. But in all cases, the veterinary surgeons responsibility is to do the best for the animal under their care.

4

VETS AND ALLIED PROFESSIONS

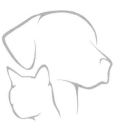

> ## KEY POINTS
>
> - Veterinary surgeons make up part of a team working to improve animal health and welfare.
>
> - Sometimes the veterinary surgeon will lead the team and sometimes they will be only part of the team.
>
> - Good communication between all members of the team is critical to success.

Vets work as part of a team of people who are all working with the animals for various reasons. These people may be qualified and well-trained or they may be keen and well-meaning amateurs. The ability to manage all of these people and be part of an integrated team is a key skill of a veterinary surgeon. Whether the veterinary surgeon is the leader of any team is a matter of context. Working with all of these team members is not, as it is unlikely that a vet will be successful working in isolation.

VETERINARY NURSES

Clients taking their pet dogs, cats, birds, reptiles and all the other animals that are kept as companions will almost certainly meet the veterinary nurses employed by the practice. In most of the world, 'veterinary nurse' is the usual term but in

USA and Canada they are referred to as 'veterinary technicians' or 'veterinary technologists'. Whatever they are called, these veterinary professionals are key to many if not all the cases being managed successfully in a practice.

The special status of veterinary nurses was recognised in the UK in 2000 in the Veterinary Surgeons Act, which allowed the nurse to carry out minor surgical procedures such as stitching wounds, removing warts or administering intravenous drugs. It would be a mistake to think that veterinary nurses are mini-vets as they have a different emphasis in their work.

"Vets repair and nurses care".

A veterinary nurse in the practice will be a force multiplier in case management. Having a skilled team member to whom the monitoring, administration of even complex treatment plans and some diagnostic testing can be delegated will allow the veterinary surgeon to work with many more animals.

In companion animal practice in many countries – in particular in the USA – the veterinary technician may take a history and perform the initial clinical examination. This will be reported to the veterinary surgeon to help them make a treatment plan as efficiently as possible. The nurse (or technician) will monitor anaesthesia after the veterinary surgeon has induced it. The veterinary surgeon may also ask the nurse to take radiographs (X-ray images) of the animal. Many veterinary nurses take far better pictures with this equipment anyway.

In addition to supporting the veterinary surgeon in treating animals, the nurse can take the lead in teaching owners about routine care of animals. In companion animal practice this may be as part of a puppy party or geriatric care examinations.

The smooth running of any practice is an important part of successful animal care. Accurate and timely recording of clinical matters will ensure that the correct treatments are given; changes in the animal's condition will be detected and acted upon before they cause further problems as a result of the assessments by the nurses.

Management of the practice may be part of the veterinary nurse's role with organizing staffing levels to ensure that there are enough people around to deliver the practice's responsibilities.

Veterinary nurses probably are most commonly employed in companion animal practices, with cats and dogs being the most frequent patients. However, in companion animal practice, all sorts of species will be seen by veterinary nurses. Another branch of practice that veterinary nurses deal with is equine practice, where they will support equine vets and be mainly based in hospitals. Nurses are found working in zoos across the world; the work is the same as for all others as regards being involved in routine treatments and vaccinations, and undertaking diagnostic tests, but vaccinating a lion cub while the mother is around will be a slightly different challenge!

EQUINE DENTIST

Many vets will work with horses to maintain their teeth in good condition. Good dental care will prevent abscesses in the jaw, allow the horse to eat well and maintain its bodyweight and muscle. Poor dental condition will cause pain and discomfort to the animal and waiting for the teeth to develop problems will make the eventual solution more difficult and expensive. Routine treatment is recommended in order to maintain the health of the horse. In order to fill a need due to the lack of equine vets or a perceived cost associated with asking a veterinary surgeon to carry out the task, equine dental technicians will carry out routine dental examinations.

The range of work that can be carried out by an equine dentist varies depending on the level of qualification and location of the dentist. In the UK there are two categories of procedures that may be carried out on a horse's mouth as written down in the legislation. Category one procedures are considered the least invasive and with the least risk associated with them. Procedures such as examining the teeth, removing points and overgrowth with a manual rasp (rasping) can be carried out by anyone whether they are qualified or not. Further qualifications in equine dentistry can be achieved. These exams are approved by DEFRA and allow the person who passes them to evaluate the horse's teeth and record dental abnormalities, remove very loose teeth and remove more attached teeth under the supervision of a veterinary surgeon. The qualified equine dentist will rasp fractured teeth and can use power instruments to rasp teeth.

Most other countries have similar models; in the USA there is legislation at state level with Hawaii only allowing veterinary surgeons to practice equine dentistry, the remaining states having differing levels of tasks that can be delegated to the equine dentist. In Australia, equine dentists are able to remove diseased teeth unlike in most other countries.

Many of these tasks can be carried out in well-behaved and particularly tolerant horses but the safety and welfare of horses may require that sedation is required. In the UK, as this is a prescription medicine, only a veterinary surgeon may prescribe and administer sedatives to calm the horse. Once the sedative drug is administered then the veterinary surgeon may choose to monitor the horse and allow the equine dentist to carry out the examination, rasping or reprofiling of the teeth in the horse. Cooperation between equine vets and well-qualified equine dentists will contribute to the welfare of horses but equally unqualified and unprofessional dentists will compromise the welfare of horses. As with nurses, a good equine dentist will allow more animals to be treated, equine teeth should be looked at every six months and it may be impossible for a veterinary surgeon to complete all these visits and the teamwork with the equine dentist gives another option. Qualified veterinary dentists, like veterinary surgeons, will be members of a professional body such as the British Association of Equine Dental Technicians or the International Association of Equine Dentistry, showing a dedication to learning and improving the practice of equine dentistry.

This area is one where the interaction between veterinary surgeons and the associated profession is at its most difficult, with many equine dentists and veterinary surgeons resenting each other's work. Australian equine dentists have been quoted as suggesting that Australian veterinary surgeons' attempts to regulate the profession in a similar manner to the UK are anti-competitive and an attempt to gain more work for veterinary surgeons. In their defence, the veterinary surgeons suggest they are trying to protect the welfare of horses. Managing these situations requires good leadership skills at a political level and at an individual level.

PREGNANCY SCANNER

Farmers are in the business of breeding animals in order to produce food for human consumption. To do this efficiently requires as much information as possible. One vital piece of information is whether an animal is pregnant or not. There are many ways to carry out pregnancy diagnosis, one of which is to use ultrasound scanners in order to find out if an animal is pregnant.

Ultrasound uses very high frequency (above 20kHz) sound-waves that humans cannot possibly hear – very good hearing can detect up to 20kHz – to produce an image on a screen. In the case of the cattle and sheep, the image will be that of the unborn animal. Information that can be gained (apart from whether the mother is pregnant) includes how old the foetus is, how many there are and what sex they are. The veterinary surgeon can work with the information to identify individual cows that need closer examination because the scanner found something that may be abnormal. The time since the last calving can also be used to look at the performance of the herd as a whole. As with most people involved in the care of animals, good communication and cooperation will get the best outcome for the owner and animals.

ARTIFICIAL INSEMINATION TECHNICIAN

Breeding of animals is a major activity of many animal keepers. Cattle, sheep, poultry and pigs are bred for food production. Dogs and horses are kept for companionship and sport. Breeding can be by mating naturally, but in order to improve the speed of genetic improvement and reproductive efficiency, artificial insemination (AI) is sometimes used. Preservation of endangered animals may be assisted by AI techniques. AI technicians are employed to carry out this procedure and inseminate animals. AI technicians will work on cattle most commonly but sheep, pigs and dogs may all be artificially inseminated. Working with the AI technician will enable the vet to improve a farm performance, preserve important genetics and improve the breed genetics.

VETERINARY PHYSIOTHERAPIST

When animals suffer an injury or have an operation there may be pain that can last for a significant length of time afterwards. Animals that are aged may suffer from diseases such as arthritis. Physiotherapy may be helpful to aid these animals. Veterinary physiotherapists will work with veterinary surgeons to help animals with amenable problems. Treatment of animals by a physiotherapist should follow a referral from a veterinary surgeon and this is recommended in most countries. Good communication between the two professionals will aid the animal as the veterinary surgeon can inform the veterinary physiotherapist with accurate information to allow the planning of a physiotherapy regime. The veterinary physiotherapist can inform the veterinary surgeon if the condition does not improve as expected and allow reassessment to determine if further treatment is required.

CASE STUDY – EQUINE PHYSIOTHERAPIST

Horses are used as sport animals and they can become lame or show a reduced ability to move, in a manner that compromises their performance in riding events. The initial diagnosis is made by a veterinary surgeon and might be that there is an injury to the back muscles such as a torn muscle. The owner might opt for rest but this might not return the horse to full performance and a course of exercise might be instituted. The veterinary surgeon may refer or, at the request of the owner, allow referral to a qualified veterinary physiotherapist. The veterinary physiotherapist will devise a number of exercises and routines that will stretch and aid the repair of these muscles. As part of these exercises, the horse might then become lame in a hind limb through twisting during one of the physiotherapist's exercise sessions. The veterinary physiotherapist will contact the original veterinary surgeon to arrange an examination of the new issue and treatment that may include stopping or altering the course of physiotherapy that has been started.

VETERINARY BEHAVIOURIST

Animal behaviour is a frequent cause of distress to owners. Dogs that destroy furniture on separation, horses that are difficult to ride and many other issues will persuade an owner to consult a veterinary surgeon. The correction of behaviour problems is almost always long-term. Some veterinary surgeons may well have an interest, the training and the expertise, as well as the time to devote to behaviour problems. But other veterinary surgeons may not have some or all of those attributes and may ask another professional to aid the owner and animal. Due to the fact that many animals will have behavioural signs in response to medical problems, responsible (non-veterinary qualified) behaviourists will require referral from a veterinary surgeon before treating an animal, and if a new condition develops during the treatment a responsible veterinary behaviourist will refer the animal back to the veterinary surgeon.

CASE STUDY – BEHAVIOURIST

A veterinary surgeon decides that a dog has separation anxiety when the owners leave home. A referral is arranged for long-term support for the dog and the owners. This involves training of both the dog and owners to minimise the anxiety and is going well until the dog starts to show aggression on being stroked around the head.

As this is a new clinical sign, the behaviourist responsibly arranges a consult with the original veterinary surgeon. Clinical examination reveals a rotten tooth, which is dealt with and the training for separation anxiety can continue as before.

ANIMAL WELFARE OFFICERS

Animal welfare officers are employed by governments and charities to monitor the welfare of animals. Their sphere of responsibility depends on whom they work for: commercial settings such as pet shops, equine yards, markets and farms might be the focus of an officer employed by a government department, while charity-employed officers may look at animals that are kept in people's homes. In both cases, the officer through the parent organisation may seek prosecution but education is usually the preferred option. Officers may give verbal advice or may refer the owner to a veterinary surgeon to allow the animal to be examined and treated as required.

Veterinary surgeons who work in private practice are not able to bring about legal sanctions on owners who may be cruel to animals, so communication with the appropriate welfare officer may bring about action that may correct the problem even if this requires prosecution. This carries with it confidentiality and ethical issues. It may be inappropriate to release a client's name to an outside party but where welfare is compromised, the balance should lie with protecting the animal. As animal cruelty, particularly to pet dogs, may indicate a possibility of domestic abuse it is probably even more important to deal with these issues as effectively as possible.

MEAT HYGIENE INSPECTORS

Many vets work in abattoirs but they do not carry out all of the inspections them-selves, they are aided by a team of inspectors. These people are employed in abattoirs to inspect carcases and ensure that all the food that leaves the slaugh-terhouse is safe to eat or fit for human consumption. Following visual inspection, the meat inspector will make a few specified cuts into the carcase in order to look at the deeper muscle and tissues, to look at lymph nodes and to look closer at any areas where they suspect there may be a problem.

Many governments include a surveillance programme to detect the appearance of disease and determine the level of disease within the population. As part of this surveillance, the inspector is looking for disease that may be passed on to the person eating the carcase; they are also looking for conditions that will look unpleasant when the meat is sold. Visual inspection of the carcase is used to detect bovine tuberculosis. Not all diseases are obvious to eye when the inspec-tion is carried out at the abattoir, with bovine spongiform encephalopathy (BSE) being an example of a disease that is monitored by testing. BSE is an infectious disease of the brain that is able to infect humans when they eat from infected cattle. There are specific controls involving the removal of the brain, spinal cord and other tissues known to be infective for this condition. Animals are also tested for the disease. This information is used by veterinary surgeons in the abattoir to make decisions about the suitability of the carcase for human consumption and by the government veterinary surgeons to advise on research and legislation priorities for the government.

Residues of medicines are not permitted in meat that is sold to the public and slaughterhouses will check with the owner of the animals that any withdrawal periods have been exceeded. To monitor adherence to the rules and ensure safety, the inspectors will take samples from some animals to try and detect medicine residues.

With all of these functions, the meat inspector liaises with a veterinary surgeon in the abattoir to protect the welfare of the animals and the safety of the food chain. The veterinary surgeon will need to have effective communication skills to allow accurate information to be relayed through the abattoir and good leadership skills to ensure that a high standard is maintained in the workplace.

PHARMACEUTICAL REPRESENTATIVES

Veterinary medicine requires the use of medicines produced by the pharmaceutical industry. These companies all have to sell their products in order to continue to exist and in order to produce more, newer and better medicines. Selling the products can be directly to the public for some medications such as flea products but many are to be prescribed by veterinary surgeons, and pharmaceutical representatives will provide information to the veterinary surgeon in practice with the correct information and allow the prescribing veterinary surgeon the ability to be properly informed.

In order to promote the medicines that the companies wish to sell, the representative will arrange meetings with clients to discuss conditions that may be helped by the medicine. The pharmaceutical representative has to comply with very strict rules in selling these medicines, with it not being permissible to advertise the medicines to the public. However, pharmaceutical companies will raise awareness of diseases in order to support sales.

Veterinary surgeons will interact with the representatives in speaking at meetings and will discuss the latest drugs. It is important the veterinary surgeon is suitably critical of the information presented in order to make properly informed decisions; this may make them very uncomfortable.

LABORATORY TECHNICIANS

Veterinary surgeons work in laboratories either as researchers or as part of a diagnostic service such as the Animal and Plant Health Agency (APHA) in the UK, or university diagnostic labs throughout the world. Technicians will carry out the routine tests in order to support the diagnosis reached by vets in post-mortem rooms and out in practice. These people will book in samples and conduct the technical procedures on the samples and report them back. Tests can involve examining faeces under a microscope to determine the presence of parasites. Blood samples can be analysed for the levels of enzymes to detect problems with internal organs. At the most sophisticated laboratories, advanced techniques such as PCR to detect DNA or MALDI – TOF (matrix-assisted laser desorption/ionization – time of flight) that will determine the type of proteins in a sample.

Laboratory technicians can work in the practice – typically this is only the case in large practices – or they can work in large commercial diagnostic laboratories. Government surveillance centres will also employ technicians. As well as using these tests to diagnose diseases, the technicians can be involved in developing the tests – validating the use of a particular test on the population of animals that are relevant to the country.

PRACTICE MANAGERS

Running a practice is a complex task: bills need to be paid on time, legislation needs to be adhered to, staff need to be managed, supplies of everything from anaesthetic gases to tea bags have to be ordered and accounts need to be sent out to clients. These and many more tasks need coordination and the larger the practice, the more complex each of the tasks becomes. Most practices will employ a manager to carry out these tasks and ensure that the practice runs efficiently. In the US, the National Council of Veterinary Economic Issues has come to the conclusion that practices that employ a manager are likely to be more efficient and this is thought to be the same all over the world.

NUTRITIONIST

The optimal performance of an animal depends in a great part on its feeding regime. Many veterinary surgeons have expertise in this and there are societies to encourage research and training in this area, such as the American College of Veterinary Nutrition. In addition to veterinary nutritionists there are professionals who will advise on feeding of many species. Nutritionists advise on the feeding of farm animals of all types, horses, zoo species and companion animals.

Probably the most common nutritional advice sought is from the farming community. The outlay of feed for animals is probably the biggest cost in producing food and the advice given either by the veterinary surgeon with an interest in nutrition or a nutritionist is invaluable in maintaining a sustainable farming business.

Nutritionists may be employed by feed companies to support their clients whether these are farmers, horse owners or companion animal owners. Others may be independent consultants working with clients in all areas and being paid by the animal owners. Nutritional advice is therefore available from many sources and the veterinary surgeon will find themselves working alongside these advisors. Some information will be less reliable than others and it is part of the job to advise the clients how to discern whether the information is factual and appropriate.

CASE STUDY – NUTRITIONIST

The farmer on a dairy farm is having problems with cows not getting up after calving and the veterinary surgeon diagnoses subclinical milk fever (low calcium in blood of cattle). The decision is made that this would be best managed by altering the feeding. A nutritionist is consulted to design a feed ration that alters the mineral balance to allow the cattle to use the calcium in the diet and in their bones effectively and reduce the milk fevers seen in the herd.

TRAINERS

Horses and dogs are probably the most common animals that are trained by their owners and many will purchase the expertise to achieve a well-trained animal. Horses are trained to jump and race, dogs are trained for showing, rescue and as assistance dogs. Other animals may be trained for filming.

In some cases, the trainer will act as a proxy for the owner such as in racehorse training where several people may own a horse and will stable it with a professional trainer in order to get that animal to a winning state. Other trainers will have the animals come to them and provide training individually or in groups.

GROOMERS

Dog grooming parlours are seen in many towns and they are owned by groomers who wash and trim the hair of dogs. As this involves the careful inspection of the dog while trimming they may well advise the owner to have skin conditions or lumps on the dog checked by a veterinary surgeon.

Some groomers may sell products that either compete with the veterinary surgeon's business or may cause harm to animals if used inappropriately, such as on the wrong species of animal or too frequently.

FIRE BRIGADE

Animals get themselves into dangerous situations and people are liable to attempt to rescue these animals, putting themselves in danger as well. In order to prevent this, fire brigades have invested in training to allow safe and effective recovery of animals that have got themselves into difficulty. In these rescue situations, the veterinary surgeon may well be called on to advise the rescue team.

Deciding that an animal is suitable for rescue, the physical state of the animal, its temperament and what the owner will require it to do after rescue all influence the decision about how the animal will be recovered from the site.

If the animal is suitable for rescue then the veterinary surgeon may assist the rescue team by giving sedative drugs to calm the animal or pain control in order to make the animal as comfortable as possible. They may also offer advice on options that are being considered in order to minimise further injuries to the animal.

It may be that the animal is so badly injured that it is wiser to euthanase the animal on site, in which case the veterinary surgeon will have to advise the fire brigade team leader that this is the case.

All rescue services have a primary aim of preserving human life, and even in animal rescue situations that still applies and the veterinary surgeon in these situations is likely to be one of a team and under the control of a primary scene commander; taking direction from that individual about when it is safe to approach the animal and what other work is being carried out at the scene and how it might impact on safety of the veterinary surgeon. Many rescues are as a result of road traffic accidents and there may be injured people, moving vehicles and other dangers to be taken into account before working with the animals.

POLICE

As a professional, the veterinary surgeon may be called upon to work with the police when animals are involved. The police have animals working in the service, such as sniffer dogs and police horses. These will need veterinary care as much as – if not more than – most other animals. The veterinary surgeon will provide routine care such as vaccination and worming. They will advise on health problems and assist in deciding whether animals are capable of carrying out their task, whether that is patrolling the streets during crowd control situations or searching for drugs in house arrests.

Police may also come across stray animals or become responsible for animals following arrests or in other circumstances during the course of their duties. They then may call upon the veterinary surgeons in the local area to assist them. The specific task carried out will depend on the situation that the animal is found in, but frequently the assessment will be of the animal's welfare and a detailed examination will be part of a potential welfare case.

ARMED FORCES

The armed forces also use animals and they will have trainers and animal care staff for the dogs and horses. These animals are used as bomb detectors, security and force protection (attack). The trainers and handlers will work in close liaison with the veterinary surgeons that work in the military, as the readiness of these animals could make a vital contribution to the security of the nation.

FARM STAFF/YARD WORKERS/KENNEL HANDS/ HANDLERS

Many animals are not looked after by the owner on a day-to-day basis as there are too many or the owner is busy managing the entire business. Staff may be employed to carry out the practical tasks of the enterprise such as cleaning animal accommodation, grooming, feeding, milking and exercising the animals. Those who carry out these tasks will have important information about the animals due to their daily contact with them. The ability to communicate well will elicit a lot of information that may be of value to a veterinary surgeon in reaching a diagnosis.

The people involved in the day-to-day care of the animals will be critical in delivering the changes required as regards treatments. More difficult for the veterinary surgeon is delivering changes in the management of the animals; the owner may specify changes but the staff will have to deliver. Probably the most effective way to ensure that the appropriate changes are made in the management of the animals is to convince the staff of the need for the changes. The ability to explain and teach the concepts underlying the changes being made will lead to greater acceptance and these management changes may well prevent further disease in the group. These may be as simple as cleaning tools between cattle foot trimming or between clipping animals, or may be fundamental changes regarding the keeping of the animals, such as moving them outside from being inside or changing from routine worming to a more risk-based approach.

CASE STUDY – FOOT TRIMMING ON FARM

On a dairy farm, lameness is an important issue for welfare and economic reasons. Lame animals will produce less milk and take longer to get pregnant again. An important member of the team is the foot trimmer, who will look at the feet of the cattle, return them to the correct shape and determine the type of problems that are most common on any individual farm. This might be the presence of damage in the white line – a structure that joins the sole and wall of the foot. This information can be used by the veterinary surgeon to determine the best treatments for the farm; more importantly, the lesions identified during the routine trimming of the cattle's feet can point to management problems in the farm that need to be corrected. In the case of white line disease, the veterinary surgeon might recommend repairs to the tracks the cattle might use. Once these changes have been made then the foot trimmer can monitor the success (or otherwise) of these changes and inform the veterinary surgeon of the change in the number of types of foot problems on the farm. This requires some form of communication and the more open these communications are, the better the outcome for the farmer and the cows on the farm.

VETERINARY SURGEONS AND OTHER PROFESSIONS

Veterinary surgeons will interact with many other professions in delivering care to the animals. In some cases the veterinary surgeon will be the leader of the team managing the care. Other situations will require the surgeon to act as a teacher to facilitate changes in management. Some situations will see the veterinary surgeon being a minor part of the team such as at a rescue situation.

People skills are critical for veterinary surgeons. These include effective communication skills, empathy and the ability to build respect, as well as listening to people and respecting their strengths and weaknesses. The veterinary surgeon will also have to demonstrate excellent professionalism, command respect and they may be required to show decisiveness and leadership.

It is important for animal welfare that all people working with the animals are working together. It is the veterinary surgeon's responsibility to ensure that happens, but *how* that occurs depends on the application of people management skills developed throughout the education of the veterinary surgeon and their further career.

5

VETS AND THE ACRONYMS

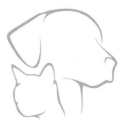

KEY POINTS

- Veterinary Surgeons use many acronyms as shorthand to speed up communication.

- Acronyms frequently refer to organisations that are important to veterinary surgeons.

- Asking for clarification of these terms will help understanding.

The veterinary profession has many acronyms associated with it and many organisations, activities and qualifications are better known by these acronyms than the full name.

THE LETTERS AFTER A NAME

Each university will award a degree and each degree is called something slightly different. These degrees all demonstrate the holder has achieved the standards required to pass an exam that demonstrates an appropriate level of knowledge and skill. To actually practice in the UK requires membership of the Royal College of Veterinary Surgeons but – except in one case (see below) – this is automatically granted on passing these exams. Upon passing, Cambridge University will award a Bachelor of Arts, Bachelor of Veterinary Medicine BA VetMB; Bristol will award a Bachelor of Veterinary Science BVSc, as will Liverpool University.

Edinburgh awards a Bachelor of Veterinary Medicine and Surgery, as does Glasgow University, although Edinburgh graduates will use the letters BVM&S while Glasgow graduates use BVMS. Nottingham awards a Bachelor of Veterinary Medicine, Bachelor of Veterinary Surgery with integrated Bachelor of Veterinary Medical Sciences, BVM BVS BVMedSc. The Royal Veterinary College in London awards a Bachelor of Veterinary Medicine, BVetMed. The University of Surrey will award a Bachelor in Veterinary Medicine and Science, BVMSci – although in this particular case, approval will need to be gained before holders of this qualification can practice as veterinary surgeons. If this approval is granted, this qualification will have the same status as those from the other universities. All of these degrees are equivalent when it comes to working as a veterinary surgeon, so a graduate from any of these universities will be able to work in any of the potential careers. Once the degree is awarded, the student becomes an MRCVS – a member of the Royal College of Veterinary Surgeons – and is allowed to practice as a veterinary surgeon.

Other courses, particularly those in the USA and Europe, will award a Doctorate in Veterinary Medicine, DVM. This is the equivalent of the awards made by the universities in the UK and to the MVB awarded by Dublin University. In the countries where these are awarded, graduates will have to register with the appropriate licensing bodies but may be eligible to register in the UK as an MRCVS as well.

Australian universities awarding a veterinary degree will award either a Bachelor of Veterinary Science and Medicine, BVMS (Murdoch University), a Bachelor of Veterinary Science, BVSc (James Cook Adelaide), or a Bachelor of Veterinary Biology/Doctor of Veterinary Medicine, BVetBiol/DVM (Melbourne and Sydney universities).

All of these confer on the holder the privilege of treating animals as long as the holder registers with the appropriate licensing body in the country where they are working, such as the Royal College of Veterinary Surgeons (RCVS) or Australian Veterinary Association (AVA).

VETERINARY ORGANISATIONS

There are many organisations that are of relevance to veterinary surgeons and students. These organisations are professional bodies that create the rules that all vets agree to adhere to. Others are bodies that represent vets in the political theatre and to the public and these may reflect relatively specialised interests within the veterinary sphere.

RCVS

Each veterinary surgeon in the world was once a veterinary student and studied at a university. Universities are not just permitted to graduate veterinary students and allow them to practise veterinary medicine on the animal belonging to a member of the public. Among many other organisations that the university has to demonstrate its quality to is the licensing body for veterinary medicine in that particular country. The Royal College of Veterinary Surgeons (RCVS) fulfils this function in the UK; in the US the American Veterinary Medical Association (AVMA) checks colleges. The Veterinary Schools Accreditation Advisory Committee (VSAAC) – which reports to the Australasian Veterinary Boards Council (AVBC) – checks colleges in Australia and New Zealand. For the European Union, the European Association of Establishments for Veterinary Education (EAEVE) carries out quality assurance for veterinary colleges. In other countries outside of these areas, local rules will apply.

What the RCVS does is assemble a team of qualified and competent inspectors. The people are generally highly qualified vets with extensive experience in veterinary education. These will look at all aspects of the life of the veterinary college. They will talk to staff and students to ensure that there is sufficient teaching staff of the correct quality and that the students are doing well. They will look at the site to ensure that the facilities are appropriate, and this includes the sporting and social facilities. This will ensure that the students have a fulfilling time at the college.

Looking at the curriculum, the RCVS team will try and determine if the students are likely to reach Day 1 competencies either through the curriculum or through ability to undertake extramural studies (EMS). Lastly, the visitors will look at the examinations carried out by the college to ensure that students will have to demonstrate an appropriate level of knowledge and skills in order to pass.

On the day of graduation the fledgling veterinary surgeon will take an oath and join the RCVS. Once this oath is taken then the student's – now the veterinary surgeon's – name is entered into the register.

THE RCVS OATH

I PROMISE AND SOLEMNLY DECLARE that I will pursue the work of my profession with integrity and accept my responsibilities to the public, my clients, the profession and the Royal College of Veterinary Surgeons, and that, ABOVE ALL, my constant endeavour will be to ensure the health and welfare of animals committed to my care.

The RCVS keeps this register of practising veterinary surgeons in the UK. In addition to the graduates of the UK veterinary colleges, graduates of colleges in European countries, graduates of commonwealth countries, graduates of AVMA-accredited programmes and those veterinary surgeons who have passed the statutory examination are also entered. The statutory examination is an examination for students that do not fit into any of the other groups but have a desire to work in the UK. It is administered by the RCVS and it confers the privilege of being able to work as a veterinary surgeon and to be independently regulated by a group of professional peers. This regulatory role is another function of the RCVS.

As a regulator, the RCVS will look into complaints made by the members of the public. As veterinary surgeons we are committed to performing our work to a very high standard. If we fail to carry out our tasks to a sufficiently high standard then the veterinary surgeons may leave themselves vulnerable to being disciplined by the RCVS. Complaints are commonly about misdiagnosis or mistreatment as the owner is unhappy with the outcome of the treatment. Almost all veterinary surgeons are carrying out clinical work to a high level, but this may not be effectively communicated to the owner. As demonstrated in Chapter 3, all diagnostic techniques and treatments come with a level of uncertainty and this needs to be communicated to the owner. Talking to clients, getting informed consent for any work carried out and discussing all the options are all very important. Poor communication with owners, other vets and the public is the main cause of most complaints, so being clear to owners is very useful. The veterinary surgeon is obliged to keep accurate records, which will aid in the management of cases and allows others to pick up the case. It also allows the RCVS to determine what actually occurred. For this reason, a lack of clinical records is considered a problem, as well as being an indication of a lack of professionalism. Professionals – particularly those in a self-regulated profession such as the veterinary profession in the UK

– are expected to be honest. This means that if a mistake occurs – and mistakes are inevitable – the person making the mistake is expected to be open about it. Trying to hide it is a matter that will attract penalties from the RCVS. It is important that the vet is open about everything that happens to the animal in order to avoid clients misunderstanding comments or issues.

Mishandling of animals by aggressive handling is also a disciplinary matter. This can occur as owners misinterpret handling techniques or if the animal is aggressive. A biting dog may not be amenable to gentle handling techniques. The safety of the vet and others may require quite tough handling, which the owner will not always appreciate. It can be difficult to explain under these probably quite emotional circumstances, but explanations should always be tried.

A particularly difficult problem for the profession and one that has caused a few high-profile cases in the veterinary press is the provision of emergency cover. The ability to provide first aid and pain relief is a core value of the profession, and failing to do so is again a disciplinary matter.

Veterinary surgeons have a privileged position in providing medicines to the public and failing to store and use these in a professional matter is considered a matter for action by the RCVS.

Being reported to the RCVS for one of these problems is a potentially highly stressful and extremely emotional event in a veterinary surgeon's life. The complaint is referred to a committee called the preliminary investigation (PI) committee. This committee will look at the evidence submitted by the complainant and by the veterinary surgeon. If the infraction is considered serious enough then the complaint is referred to the disciplinary committee for further investigation. This committee is made up of both vets and non-vets (referred to as laypeople) to give representation of both the veterinary viewpoint and that of the client.

The committee exists to maintain public confidence in the veterinary profession and so must take all complaints seriously but must also be fair to all concerned. This can lead to long and detailed discussions before a decision is reached. If the veterinary surgeon is found guilty of a breach of the code then they will be sanctioned. However, this can take many forms: sanctions can be advice to avoid further problems or mandatory retraining on specific or general issues. If there are medical or other administrative issues then these may have to be addressed and failure to do so will lead to more severe penalties. The committee can also recommend that the vet is removed from the register – and therefore not allowed to practice – for a period of time.

The RCVS is not only a punitive organisation but also it awards honours to those that – in the view of the members and the various committees – have contributed significantly to the profession. This can be done through submitting a thesis or contributing to learning for prolonged periods and this allows the veterinary surgeon to use the term 'fellow' in place of 'member' so they become fellows of the Royal Veterinary College (FRCVS).

Other countries also have similar arrangements, with the United States having state boards that will deal with registration and any complaints about vets practising in the state. Australia has a similar system, with each of the states having its own veterinary practitioners' board. In New Zealand, an organisation similar to the RCVS – the Veterinary Council of New Zealand – works to protect the public interest by ensuring that vets practice to a high standard.

WVA

The veterinary profession is represented by a number of bodies on matters such as political changes that will have a bearing on veterinary surgeons in their practice. At a world level, the World Veterinary Medicine Association (WVA) is an overarching body that is made up of membership from countries' professional associations. The WVA tries to promote the interests of veterinary medicine, animal welfare and public health throughout the world.

Organisations that are members of the WVA include the British Veterinary Association (BVA), the American Veterinary Medical Association (AVMA), the Australian Veterinary Association (AVA) and the Federation of Veterinarians of Europe (FVE). These members all contribute to the discussions about the future of veterinary medicine.

BVA

The British Veterinary Association (BVA) represents its membership of veterinary surgeons and veterinary nurses. Its membership is roughly about 50 per cent of the veterinary surgeons registered with the RCVS and about 80 per cent of the vets working in the UK. The BVA works to represent the industry in the UK and has consulted and lobbied on a diverse range of issues. These include topics such as the use of aversive training devices, tail docking dogs, antibiotic resistance, education of vets and bovine TB. Through online forums and meetings, the opinions of the veterinary profession are collected on any of these matters and reported to government and other interested parties.

The BVA also delivers training to vets so that they can keep their skills up-to-date on all areas that might be required, from management to backyard bird treatment.

The BVA cooperates with the Kennel Club to administer dog health schemes. These schemes are in place to allow breeders of dogs to make informed decisions about whether to breed from the dogs. The schemes look at hip dysplasia (hip problems), elbow dysplasia (elbow growth problems), hereditary eye disease and chiari/syringomyelia problems (deformities of the spinal column).

AVMA

THE AVMA OATH

Being admitted to the profession of veterinary medicine, I solemnly swear to use my scientific knowledge and skills for the benefit of society through the protection of animal health and welfare, the prevention and relief of animal suffering, the conservation of animal resources, the promotion of public health, and the advancement of medical knowledge. I will practice my profession conscientiously, with dignity, and in keeping with the principles of veterinary medical ethics. I accept as a lifelong obligation the continual improvement of my professional knowledge and competence.

The American Veterinary Medicine Association (AVMA) has the same aims as the BVA. It supports the veterinarians working in the United States by advocating on a number of issues such as soring horses (making the feet painful to produce a specific walking style), keeping exotic animal species, indigenous species conservation, the ability to prescribe drugs and food safety and supporting farming in the United States. Due to the way that the United States is organized politically, it also represents veterinarians on issues that are legislated at a state level rather than a federal level.

It also has a charitable arm, the American Veterinary Medical Foundation, and this supports initiatives from disaster relief, public education and research as well as student support.

In addition to the advocacy and charitable work carried out by the AVMA, the organisation provides accreditation for educational establishments. This inspection is voluntary for the colleges that contribute to the programme. To practice in the United States requires a licence from the state licensing board and to get this licence requires proof of attending a suitable course. Graduation from a veterinary college accredited by the AVMA is one of the criteria that the licensing boards use to determine the suitability of the applicant. Accreditation is carried out in a similar manner to the visits by the RCVS in the UK. The colleges are inspected for their ability to graduate veterinary surgeons with the skills that are required. The research performance of the institution is also evaluated.

OTHER ACCREDITING BODIES

In Australia and New Zealand the accreditation of colleges is carried out by the Veterinary Schools Accreditation Advisory Committee (VSAAC), which reports to the Australasian Veterinary Boards Council (AVBC). European Veterinary Colleges are also accredited by the European Association of Establishments for Veterinary Education (EAEVE). Frequently colleges may have accreditations from the RCVS, AVMA, EAEVE and AVBC. When choosing a college, many students will have these accreditations in mind, as they will affect where they can practice after graduation.

TABLE 5.1 A few of the specialist veterinary organisations. There are many more!

Acronym	Full name
BCVA	British Cattle Veterinary Association
AABP	American Association of Bovine Practitioners
SPVS	Society of Practising Veterinary Surgeons
BSAVA	British Small Animal Veterinary Association
GVS	Goat Veterinary Society
BEVA	British Equine Veterinary Association
SVS	Sheep Veterinary Society
SAVMA	Student American Veterinary Medicine Association
AVS	Association of Veterinary Students
VPMA	Veterinary Practice Management Association

SPECIALIST ORGANISATIONS

The BVA is supported by many smaller veterinary organisations. These are groups of veterinary surgeons that have an interest in a specific species such as cattle or a specific discipline such as dermatology. In a similar manner, the AVMA has similar specialist organisations allied to it. Both the AVMA and the BVA use these organisations to give a more informed opinion from policies and statements produced.

The organisations listed in Table 5.1 will sponsor professional education and research in the areas of interest for its members. The SVS is interested in how to control the intestinal parasites of sheep and minimise resistance to the treatments available. Through Petsavers, the BSAVA promotes research into kidney disease in cats and improving pain control in small animals. The BCVA and the AABP have sponsored research into the foot health of cattle, particularly dairy cattle.

OTHER IMPORTANT ORGANISATIONS

VDS

The Veterinary Defence Society (VDS) is a UK-specific organisation and provides insurance cover for veterinary surgeons in the UK. This is a mutual insurance company set up by veterinary surgeons in the UK and covers most of the vets in the UK. In the UK, as in most countries, it is becoming increasingly common for veterinary surgeons to be sued and the VDS helps to defend against claims. It also helps represent defendants in disciplinary cases in front of the RCVS. There are analogous organisations throughout the world, such as the Veterinary Defence Association for Australia.

Defra

All countries have a government department that regulates the agriculture industry. In the UK this is Defra – the Department for Environment Farming and Rural Affairs. In the United States it is the USDA – United States Department of Agriculture – that regulates farming. In Australia the relevant body is the Department of Agriculture. New Zealand has the Ministry for Primary Industries (MPI) and all of these organisations will see rules that affect veterinary surgeons directly, such as specifying testing for specific diseases. Where the government sponsors disease eradication – such as bovine viral diarrhoea virus as carried out in Scotland, Ireland, Scandinavia and other parts of Europe – this will directly affect the veterinary and farming industries. For veterinary surgeons that do not have farming clients, these departments may still have an impact as some clients will have pet sheep, pet pigs and pet llamas, as well as other animals. These will still come under the regulations set out by the farming department.

For those in companion or equine practice with no clients having pet farm animals, these departments will also deal with the export and import of pet animals and horses.

These departments also incorporate the government veterinary services. The UK agency is called the Animal and Plant Health Agency (APHA) and each country has similar agencies with similar but not identical functions.

OIE

It was recognised decades ago that the control of many diseases would require coordination at an international level. In 1924, the Office International des Epizooties (World Organisation for Animal Health, OIE) was set up as a body that, with the agreement of 24 countries, would act in this manner. The OIE now acts as a reference, with government vets reporting to the organisation the number and type of diseases within the borders of their countries. These reports are collated and then outbreaks can be monitored. This is in order to ensure that the disease situation across the world is transparent. The OIE collates and disseminates scientific information to aid disease control and encourage cross border cooperation in disease control. It contributes to food safety by setting out the standards that should be adhered to if trade in animals is to be carried out. Critical to this in any country or region is the presence of a strong veterinary service, whether that is government- or privately funded, and the OIE supports the provision of these services where required. It also tries to promote animal welfare by setting standards that have been accepted by the member countries, such as standards for stray dog control or the killing of farmed fish.

The original 24 states that formed the OIE have now expanded to encompass 180 countries with permanent membership. The government department in each country sends a representative to report on animal health concern, the UK is represented by the chief veterinary officer and the United States by an administrator of USDA, and all 180 countries send similarly qualified veterinary representatives in order to work on disease control.

VMD

Veterinary surgeons have a wide array of drugs with which to work, but to allow them to be administered to animals or sold through vets, pet stores, farmers cooperatives or any other shop, it is important that the medicines are safe. The responsibility lies with the Veterinary Medicines Directorate (VMD). The VMD will accept applications from companies to allow the sale of veterinary medicines in the UK and veterinary experts at the VMD will consider the evidence presented and make a decision to allow the medicine onto the market. This evidence will come from scientific studies demonstrating the safety of the medicine so that the public can be assured that any problems will not be worsened by the use of the medicine. How well the drug works at its stated purpose is also examined, this means that when the vet uses it to treat a specific condition it is likely to be successful. As vets are concerned with food production as well as treating animals to get them better, the effect on humans is also considered. The presence of the medicine in meat, milk and eggs is studied with safe limits for people being established. Following detailed studies a maximum residue limit (MRL) is set for presence in human foodstuffs. The rate at which the medicine is removed from meat, milk or eggs is then used to determine how long the time period between administration and slaughter, milking or egg collection should be left. This is marked on all publicity and bottles, packets or leaflets sent out in relation to the product. Both the famer and the vet have a responsibility to ensure that any animal treated has no medicine residues that can compromise health. Although the withdrawal periods are set by the VMD, there are many circumstances where the prescribing vet will alter the length of time; for example, the veterinary surgeon can lengthen the period of time that an animal will have to be kept out of food production. The MRL is a minimum time period and high dosing, more frequent doses and longer periods of treatment will affect the withdrawal period.

The VMD also monitors the performance of the drugs after marketing. The VMD monitors the level of adverse events that occur due to the use of a specific medicine. This uses the yellow form – an adverse reaction reporting form. When a vet suspects that a problem has occurred and that it may be due to the administration of the medicine or a microchip, then details of the administered product, the person who carried out the work, the animal or group along with the reasons for treating the animals are sent to the VMD. These reports are collated and if a trend is detected then the product may have its licence altered to account for these problems or may be withdrawn from the market completely. In recent years, a vaccine against an important cattle disease was removed as systems in many countries including Germany, New Zealand and the UK were alerted to the association with vaccinating cattle for bovine viral diarrhoea and calves developing a syndrome associated with unexpected and severe bleeding that lead to the death of most affected calves. With cooperation from the manufacturer, the vaccine was withdrawn and cases reduced markedly. To act in this manner, the VMD needs evidence to make the decision and, as some products are sold outside the veterinary surgeries, the reporting system is not used; instead complaints are made direct to the manufacturer. For example, a company selling flea control products containing permethrin, which can cause poisoning when applied to cats. The cats twitch uncontrollably, have a fever and can have seizures, all of which are distressing to both animal and owner, and can be fatal in some cases. The company chose to replace the active ingredient in the product following campaigns by members of the public and International Cat Care.

In addition to looking for adverse effects associated with the animals, the safety to humans has to be considered. This is mainly monitoring that no traces of the medicines used on the animals remain when they are eaten. Through an associated organization, the Veterinary Residues Committee (VRC), the animals that are used to produce food are monitored for residual traces of medicine. All animals slaughtered (sheep, cattle, pigs, poultry, fish, rabbits and other game), as well as milk, honey and eggs are liable to be sampled. The number of samples taken is huge, but the number of samples that are found to contain levels of medicine that is too high is very small.

Detection of medicines in the samples will result in penalties to the producer. These are usually financial and may involve other agencies inspecting the farm of origin. In most cases, it is an inadvertent problem due to poor communication between veterinary staff and farm staff, or poor recordkeeping on farm leading to the wrong animal being milked or sent to the abattoir. A change to the way the medicine is administered to the animal may result in it taking longer to clear the medicine than indicated on any labels. Out of date medicines may be removed from the animal's body at a different rate depending on changes that occur after the expiry date.

Unauthorised medicines that come from sources such as overseas-based internet sites may not be what is indicated on the label, leading to failures. Horses are a particular problem as one of the most common painkillers used in horse medicine – phenylbutazone or bute – renders that animal unsuitable for human consumption. In Europe, all horses have a passport and not recording that the horse has been treated and therefore is not to be put in the food chain can lead to residue limit failures. As in a lot of issues in veterinary medicine, accurate records will assist in stopping these problems. Communicating these issues to owners is an important part of the veterinary surgeons task when working with farmers and horse owners.

The safety of people and animals is not the limit of the VMD's interest. Environmental safety is also considered. Some of the methods used to administer treatments can lead to potential contamination of watercourses. Dipping sheep with organo-phosphates is a particular example in the UK. Fish farming is an industry where environmental damage is a particular concern as the medicines may be administered directly into the water. Although this water is contained, disposal must be considered, as well as the potential for the inadvertent escape of treated water.

NOAH

Another organisation that is involved in the veterinary medicine industry is the National Office of Animal Health (NOAH). This body represents the manufacturers of medicines to the government and the public. It acts to promote responsibility in manufacturing and sale of veterinary medicines, and it promotes the benefits of medicines to the public.

For a veterinary surgeon, NOAH produces the compendium of datasheets every year. A datasheet is all of the relevant information regarding a particular product. This includes the name the product is sold under, the active ingredient, its dosing instructions, what form it takes and withdrawal periods, along with any other legal information required. The compendium collects all of the updated sheets and is published yearly providing an immensely useful resource for vets.

FSA

The Food Standards Agency (FSA) in the UK is responsible for the safety of food, labelling and enforcement of the relevant laws. Many vets are employed in slaughterhouses, checking that the activities in slaughterhouses are up to standard. The equivalent in the US is the Food Safety and Inspection Service. Australia has a meat inspection system, the Australian Export Meat Inspection Service (AEMIS) that works alongside the internal meat inspection regime to allow export to other countries, with veterinarians providing quality assurance to the system.

RSPCA/SSPCA

The first national animal charity created was the Royal Society for the Prevention of Cruelty to Animals (RSPCA). The RSPCA works to reduce animal cruelty in the

UK and has had a huge amount of influence on legislation in the UK. Initially the RSPCA started with the main focus on horses, but now encompasses all animals. In order to assist farm animal welfare, the RSPCA also works as part of a farm assurance scheme – Freedom Food – to help the public buy food that is produced in a manner that they would consider acceptable. The RSPCA employs veterinary surgeons to treat animals where the owner is not able to pay for treatment. It will also pay for immediate emergency treatment (IET) at private veterinary practices. What constitutes IET and the level of treatment available is always under review and, like all charities, is dependent on the amount of money donated by members of the public.

The RSPCA does not operate in Scotland and in its place is the Scottish Society for the Prevention of Cruelty to Animals (SSPCA) that has an analogous role. Both of these organisations will prosecute where required: the RSPCA through private prosecutions and the SSPCA through the prosecutor fiscal office (the Scottish government department that prosecutes criminal cases). In addition, SSPCA inspectors have the authority to search premises and seize animals. An interesting and valuable initiative that the SSPCA carries out is an education programme that is part of the Scottish curriculum in primary school.

Organisations analogous to these exist in all countries throughout the world. The staff involved in these organisations work hard to reduce cruelty and improve the standard of life for all animals.

OTHER ACRONYMS THAT ARE IN USE

EMS

Students studying to be veterinary students are enrolled in an intensive course with lots of studying that is required in the course. In addition to this and in order to expand the student practical experience and expose the student to a variety of experiences are extra mural studies (EMS) or seeing practice. Students in the UK and Australia are required as part of the studies to complete 38 weeks in total (for the RCVS); Australian veterinary colleges use the RCVS model for their students in order to ensure accreditation. For the RCVS this is split into 12 weeks of learning about how animals are kept (animal husbandry) and 26 weeks of clinical placements with veterinary surgeons in a variety of types of practice.

Veterinary students studying at American or European colleges are not required to undertake EMS, but many students do so anyway as it is a valuable way to gain relevant experience.

Many varieties of EMS experiences are available and looking at websites will reveal marine mammal rescue courses, primate rehabilitation courses, zoo animal care, safari capture courses, equine surgery and small animal vaccination clinics. The choice of what to do is ultimately up to the student, but these placements should be entered into with the view that they will aid the learning and aid the student in their future career. At an early stage in any career, and particularly in veterinary medicine, it is important that the basic knowledge, reasoning skills and practical skills are well embedded. These can be from understanding how cattle are fed and how horses are kept clean and exercised to blood sampling in sheep, cattle, cats and dogs. Getting these skills well-practised will be immensely valuable to vets no matter what area they finally work in. Other more specialised courses and experiences can be inspirations to the student for a future career.

CPD/CE

The training of a veterinary surgeon does not stop at graduation, with vets expected to complete ongoing training throughout their career. This is referred to as continuous professional development (CPD) in the UK and Australia and continuous education (CE) in the US. The RCVS expects its members to undertake 105 hours of CPD over three years, an average of 35 hours per year. In the US, this is decided at the state level but most states require similar levels of training for veterinary surgeons. Australian veterinary surgeons are obliged to pursue CPD worth 60 points every three years. Different activities attract different numbers of points with clinical reviews getting up to ten points for completing one. New Zealand has a very similar system.

The range of activities that veterinary surgeons undertake to comply with their responsibilities as members of their professional bodies is huge. These can be attendance at lectures or seminars, they may go to wet labs and undertake practical training. They may also present to colleagues at large seminars or informal clinic-based groups. The preparation of papers for publication is also a valid CPD activity, as is reading some of the thousands of articles and papers produced by colleagues every year.

Activities that contribute to the continuous training are expected to be relevant to the career of the veterinary surgeon. The RCVS has adopted a definition of CPD as 'the systematic maintenance, improvement and broadening of knowledge and skills and the development of personal qualities necessary for the execution of professional and technical duties throughout the member's working life'. This means that a vet working with farm animals might undertake training on a specific disease or on the economics of practice, a veterinary surgeon working with cats might study behaviour in cats. For all of the associations regulating veterinary surgeons, the decision about what CPD is and should be is left to the individual veterinary surgeon.

PDP

The first few years of the graduate's career are critical in getting the individual off to a great start. Instilling a good approach to learning as a professional is a key component of a new graduate's path to becoming a skilled professional. To aid this, graduates working in the UK are asked to complete a professional development phase (PDP). This encourages veterinary graduates to think about their performance in areas such as clinical skills and communications, and provides the evidence base for any methods of work that the veterinary surgeon undertakes.

PDR

A relatively new development in the UK is an online recording system for veterinary surgeons to record the number of CPD hours that they have undertaken. This professional development record (PDR) can be used to monitor and compare the ongoing training that veterinary surgeons have to complete.

SOAP

Recording a patient's information is very important when multiple people are involved in the care, when looking back to determine what happened and formulating a plan. Having a structured way to do this is very helpful and one way to do this is using the SOAP approach. This breaks down the thought process into four steps:

1. Subjective – where the complaint is documented such as coughing or lameness.

2. Objective – this is followed by objective measures such as temperature or heart rate. The three most common objective measures are sometimes referred to as TPR – temperature, pulse (heart rate) and respiratory rate.

3. Assessment is the next step with a diagnosis or list of possible diagnoses.

4. Plan – the previous steps will lead to a plan being developed and this is what will be done to the patient either to advance the diagnosis or to complete the treatment of the patient.

Other ways of formulating the patient records are used and each veterinary surgeon may use a slightly different style. The important part is that the information is accurate and easy to read by another veterinary surgeon who may become involved in the case.

PICO

Evidence-based medicine is an increasingly important part of veterinary medicine and the ability to formulate a useful question is part of that. PICO is an attempt to help the veterinary surgeon develop these questions. As with SOAP, it represents a structure to think through.

1. Population, patients, or participants – what are the relevant patients? (For example, aged dogs.)

2. Intervention – what are we actually going to do to these patients? (Such as chondroitin sulphate administration.)

3. Control – what are we comparing the response to? Is it no treatment or to a painkilling treatment?

4. Outcome – what difference does it make to the patient? Ideally this should be an ability to walk better rather than measuring the presence of a product in the blood.

By doing this thought process, the veterinary surgeon will be able to become more refined in their thinking and get better answers to client questions or identify where the information is lacking in the wider scientific community.

MEDICAL TERMS

The veterinary profession is filled with acronyms and similar word structures. Some are associated with diseases such as BSE (bovine spongiform encephalopathy – the cause of mad cow disease) or FMD (foot and mouth disease). Other cattle diseases include BVD (bovine viral diarrhoea) and RSV (respiratory syncytial virus). In the equine world we have CEMO (contagious equine metritis) and EIA (equine infectious anaemia). Pigs can have PRRS (porcine reproductive and respiratory syndrome) or PMWS (post-weaning multi-systemic wasting syndrome). Dogs can get AIHA (autoimmune haemolytic anaemia) and cats can get FIV (feline immunodeficiency virus). The list is extensive and growing, but reading and asking about the diseases will help with your understanding.

SUMMARY

There are so many acronyms that are used between veterinary surgeons when discussing cases and issues. They are used because they facilitate rapid communication between people who know what they mean. Be looking at these acronyms and explaining what they mean, I hope to have given you an insight into different facets of the veterinary profession.

6

VETERINARY CAREERS

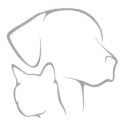

The veterinary degree is a high quality science degree and opens up the path to a number of careers that may not have previously been considered. Although the central skill of most vets is treating animals, they can use the scientific skills gained through the training at university to work in other areas. Not all of these will be working with animals directly and some who qualify may go off to work in fields with no animal contact at all. Changes in the veterinary world may result in fewer positions in practices working with the public and treating their animals. This means that applicants to veterinary degree courses need to accept that they may have to consider alternatives to the traditional veterinary career. The careers discussed in this chapter are some of the options available, and the veterinary surgeons who fulfil these roles today find them very satisfying.

GOVERNMENT VETERINARY SURGEON

The government of any country needs to set out legislation in order to protect its citizens. This legislation may be to ensure that food is safe to eat or to protect the consumer from fraudulent products. Legislation will protect the welfare of animals by ensuring that the standards of animal keeping are met within the country. The government also has a responsibility to monitor the spread of disease and influence the research priorities of the government.

When working with the government, veterinary surgeons will bring their expertise to help develop government policy. This has to be based on a good understanding of disease within the country and the science that underlies control of the disease.

As part of this, the surveillance of diseases is a government responsibility. This may involve the veterinary surgeons working either with or as epidemiologists to understand the pattern of diseases. This data may come from the pathology labs, on-farm testing or specifically commissioned research studies. Surveillance can be passive or active; these have differing roles in adding to the knowledge of animal health in a particular country. Using these approaches has detected the emergence of new diseases such as psoroptes in cattle entering the UK and the Schmallenberg virus in Europe. The identification of these new diseases allows the government to assist in controlling them and reduces the time they circulate in the animal population before appropriate control measures are applied. This method of disease detection relies on a well-designed and effective sampling system that depends on the submission of dead animals or diagnostic samples with trained pathologists and laboratory staff. The experience of these individuals will provide a diagnosis for the submitting farmer or veterinary surgeon. If a diagnosis cannot be reached – despite all the testing and training – then this could suggest that a new disease is emerging.

Well-designed studies may be commissioned by the government in order to iden-tify the size of a specific problem. Many diseases are studied to find out how many animals are affected in the population (prevalence); this is used by many organisations to decide whether they should commit resources to dealing with the disease. For governments the diseases that might be of interest will be those that have legal or human health implications such as bovine virus diarrhoea (BVD) in the UK, or West Nile virus in the USA. The decisions about whether to use the targeted active surveillance or work with the data from the intake from the passive collection of data is a constant challenge for the veterinary surgeons working within government.

Government vets will also be involved in welfare work and developing the legislation that all keepers of animals have to comply with. In conjunction with developing the legislation (alongside other stakeholders), the government veterinary surgeons will be involved in developing codes of practice to aid animal-keepers in staying within the law.

Medicines have to be licensed and veterinary surgeons will be involved in this as well, through working at organisations such as the Veterinary Medicines Directorate (VMD) in the UK, the Office of New Animal Drug Evaluation in the USA or the Australian Pesticides and Veterinary Medicines Authority. In addition to approving the sale of drugs, these organisations will monitor the safety of the medicines and consider altering or removing their authorization should a problem arise.

COMPANION VETERINARY SURGEON

When thinking about veterinary surgeons, most people will picture a vet in a white coat, carrying a stethoscope and examining a dog. These veterinary surgeons will work in specialised buildings – veterinary surgeries or practices – and will term themselves 'small animal vets' or 'companion vets'.

All animals that people keep as companions or pets will be treated by small animal veterinary surgeons. This will range from dogs and cats – which have been domesticated and companions for thousands of years – to animals that have more recently been used as companion animals such as degus, Madagascan hissing cockroaches, snakes of various species, bearded dragons, varieties of tarantula and many more species and varieties.

During a working day, the companion vet will examine animals during consultations. The time allowed can be very different depending on the veterinary practice policy in place. Consultations can range in length from five minutes to 30 minutes and this can put enormous pressure on the veterinary surgeon. Within these consultations, the animals will have to be examined and a diagnosis reached to decide on a treatment plan. Communicating the findings to the client who owns the animal must be done in an appropriate manner. If the diagnosis is straightforward then the time limit may be reasonable but in complex cases it will frequently take more time than allowed and the veterinary surgeon will take longer to complete a list of appointments. Vaccinations also are carried out during consultations; although these are perceived to be simple they may uncover a host of problems. When dealing with a predominantly cat and dog companion animal population, administering vaccinations may be the most common treatment administered and it may be one of the most important. The challenge is maintaining the attention to ensure that nothing is missed. The intellectual challenge associated with these consultations may be limited in comparison to the consultations that the veterinary student would experience at university.

Companion animal veterinary surgeons can be a small business owner; the number of vets working in the practice can range from one veterinary surgeon (the owner) to many veterinary surgeons. Owners of practices may term themselves partners, directors or owners depending on the manner in which they have set up the business. The income that these veterinary surgeons take home is directly related to the success of the business. The directors will also employ veterinary surgeons on a salary basis.

Another employment option for veterinary surgeons is to work for corporate practices such as Banfield and VCA in the US and CVS, Companion Care and Vets4pets in the UK. These are companies with boards of directors and all the associated structure of many other companies; these have varied business models and offer employment terms that some veterinary surgeons will find suitable.

Companion animal veterinary surgeons may well decide to concentrate on specific animals; for example, deciding that cats are the only animals that they wish to work with. The practices they start may be built with that animal in mind – with cat-friendly waiting rooms in feline exclusive practices that have cubby holes for cat baskets to be stored in while waiting for appointments. The veterinary surgeon may well take further advanced training in the animal(s) the practice specialises in as well.

Veterinary surgeons are notorious for working long hours. The exact time that a veterinary surgeon may be expected to work in a practice varies by the place of work. A working week will consist of daily appointments, operating during the day and evening consultation sessions. Emergencies and unexpected problems will alter the pattern of the day and may well extend well into the night. Emergencies can be anything from road traffic collisions, animals giving birth or other more complex medical conditions such as a diabetic coma. This can put pressure on the family life of the veterinary surgeon as meals will often be late and events can be cancelled at last minute.

PRACTICE OWNERSHIP

There are a number of ways that practices can be owned and managed.

Sole trader

A single veterinary surgeon is responsible for running the practice. They may employ other people to work for them including other veterinary surgeons. The owner is responsible for all the debts in the business and is paid from the profits of the business.

Partnership

The practice is owned by a number of veterinary surgeons who share the profits and the debts from the business. They can employ other staff to work for them.

Company

All the other types of business are usually owned by veterinary surgeons but a newer type is a limited company. These can be owned by anyone who can buy shares and the profits are split among the shareholders. While a practice owned by a veterinary surgeon can place animal health and welfare ahead of money, many fear that shareholder-owned operations will not.

FARM ANIMAL VETERINARY SURGEON

Veterinary surgeons provide a valuable input to the agricultural community and many veterinary surgeons will work solely with farmers and farm animals. The most common species that farm animal vets will work with are ruminants (cattle and sheep) but other species may be dealt with less commonly.

Unlike companion animal veterinary surgeons who generally ask the clients to bring the animals to their places of work, farm animal veterinary surgeons will visit the animals at the farm. Some exceptions to this exist, such as bringing ewes to the practice in order to aid them in giving birth (lambing the ewe or carrying out a caesarean section). The distance between farms can be many miles and require significant travel times. In the UK, which has farms relatively close together, a busy day may see the veterinary surgeon travelling 100 miles a day or more. Where the farms are more widely distributed, such as in Australia and parts of the USA, vets may see even greater time spent driving to farms.

Once on the farm, the veterinary surgeon may be faced with many issues. Emergencies that the surgeon may face include calving or lambing difficulties and there is the additional complication of operating on the farm, rather than in a surgery. Other emergencies may be when the gases from the rumen (first stomach compartment) of ruminants cannot escape. Rapid relief may be required to save the animal. The relief of the animal is only part of the work, as the affected animal is almost certainly part of a larger group. In order to prevent further problems, it may be necessary to work with the farmer to prevent further problems.

The traditional role of the farm animal veterinary surgeon was seen as providing this support in treating animals for disease. If there were a lung disease (calf pneumonia) then the veterinary surgeon would arrive to treat all the animals and provide further treatments as required. As farming has changed and the economic understanding of the costs of diseases has improved, the interaction between farmers and veterinary surgeons has changed. The emphasis has moved from reducing the impact of disease by rapid treatment to preventing disease and adding value to the farming business. Controlling disease on farms is also a core skill of the farm veterinary surgeon. Whether this is parasite control on sheep farms or diarrhoea control in calves, the presence of disease may have a severe financial impact and advice aimed at removing the disease may be beneficial. Improving the performance may be accomplished by conducting fertility examinations of the cattle in the herd and working out where the limitations in the herd are. This can be then used to improve the performance, leading to a successful herd.

Although disease control at a national level is coordinated by governments, the delivery of testing and monitoring may be done by privately employed veterinary surgeons. Bovine tuberculosis (TB) is a disease of cattle that can infect humans and is legally controlled by governments. Surveillance for the presence of disease is contracted out either to companies or private veterinary surgeons. The precise model is always under review as debate occurs about where the costs of removing disease are apportioned. Historically in the UK, tuberculosis testing has been carried out by the veterinary surgeon who treats the livestock on the farm. Other diseases that government veterinary surgeons and private veterinary surgeons might cooperate in dealing with include foot and mouth disease and bovine spongiform encephalopathy.

The time commitment for farm vets, as with companion animal veterinary surgeons, is substantial – emergencies, driving and evening meetings as well as a substantial requirement to complete paperwork conspire to ensure long days. The pressure on family and social life can be immense. In addition to this, the work can consist of long periods where routine straightforward tasks are required of the veterinary surgeon; many vets regard TB testing (although an important task) as a routine and fairly boring procedure. This may lead to farm vets becoming disillusioned with the routine nature of these tasks.

MIXED PRACTICE VETERINARY SURGEON

James Herriot wrote as a mixed practice veterinary surgeon. Veterinary surgeons who will work with any species are becoming less common as specialisation and the economic realities of veterinary medicine start to change the employment of veterinary surgeons. The mixed practice veterinary surgeon may start the day looking at cats, dogs and other companion animals in consultations, the rest of the day may involve working with farm animals of all species as well as horses, donkeys and all of the animals that people keep. Additionally they may be called upon to treat the wildlife of the area.

This type of employment is more common in rural areas. The distance and low population make it unlikely that specialised practices can set up in these areas.

Some practices will employ staff to fill specific needs for their clients. Although the business will be prepared to meet the needs of any animal, it will employ veterinary surgeons to work as companion, farm or equine vets.

EQUINE VETERINARY SURGEON

Some veterinary surgeons will specialise in the treatment of a specific species. They may wish to work with cats or dogs but the original area where this single-species approach occurred was in the treatment of horses. This is one of the traditional career paths associated with veterinary medicine and the traditional model of training veterinary surgeons is associated with teaching the treatment of horses along with cattle and dogs.

The work carried out by an equine veterinary surgeon during a routine day is similar in many ways to a companion animal veterinary surgeon, while other parts of the job will resemble that of a farm animal veterinary surgeon. Routine tasks will include administering vaccinations to the horses under their care and examining them for a variety of conditions.

Horses have fulfilled a large number of functions in their association with people: they have been war machines, companions, sporting animals and agricultural implements providing power. Horses still act in all these capacities in many parts of the world. Most equine veterinary surgeons will work with either sport horses or with companion animals.

Where the animals are sporting, the performance of the animals is paramount. Horses will be asked to race or jump to the limits of their ability and occasionally beyond. Many things — including lameness and problems with airways as well as general unfitness — can limit performance. In companion horses used for general hacking, the problems are often associated with overfeeding and unfitness.

An important and growing part of equine medicine is the care of geriatric animals. As more animals are kept as pets, more are living to an old age. Equine veterinary surgeons are increasingly involved in working with owners to care for older animals.

Equine veterinary surgeons will work in practices but they will also visit horses wherever they are stabled. Like farm animal veterinary surgeons, this will require a great deal of time travelling between cases.

PIG VETERINARY SURGEON

Some farming enterprises have grown to be multinational in size and are worth large amounts of money. This means that the consequences of poor advice will have a greater impact. Where the company is involved in pyramid breeding then the impact of decisions made will affect pig farms across the world.

Veterinary surgeons working for the pig industry can work as part of a practice as with most other vets; they may be independent consultants who will work for many farms and companies or they may work for a pig producer, with working hours being dependent on which route the veterinary surgeon takes. Some vets may be asked to visit pig units all over the world and fly regularly to these units.

Pig veterinary surgeons will be involved in giving advice to farmers. This can range from how pigs and people come onto the farm to disinfection of the housing after pigs have left. Pig farms are some of the most biosecurity conscious in the agricultural industry. People are not allowed on if they have worked with other pigs in the past three days and even then may be asked to shower before entering the unit. Deliveries of feed and animals are not allowed on site, with loading bays being located at a peripheral part of the farm, away from the housing or fields where the pigs are kept. Pigs are very efficient at growing but this requires careful management. The veterinary surgeon working with pigs will advise on how to manage the breeding animals to ensure that they are as productive as possible; working with growing pigs will involve looking at environmental conditions in order to make the pigs grow as quickly as possible. In addition they will work with farmers to prevent and eliminate disease through vaccination and rapid diagnosis and treatment, as might be expected from any veterinary surgeon.

POULTRY VETERINARY SURGEON

Like pigs, poultry farming for food production has developed into an industry that for some companies spans countries, and veterinary surgeons have specialised in giving advice to these companies. With the integration of the whole food chain from feed companies to the final slaughtering of the bird, poultry veterinary surgeons can have a major impact on the efficiency, health and welfare of poultry farms all over the world.

The work carried out by poultry veterinary surgeons has many similarities to the work of a pig veterinary surgeon. There is an emphasis on biosecurity aimed at stopping the introduction of disease onto a farm through managing the visitors so they do not cause an increased risk to the farm to vaccination of the flock in order to stop the spread of disease.

Accurate disease diagnosis is also, as might be expected, an important part of the services supplied to clients. In flock health situations, the diagnosis might be reached by a combination of post-mortem examination and examining data such as egg production records, water and feed consumption and environmental records such as temperature and light levels. The rapid diagnosis will minimise any loss but – as is becoming recognised across all of agriculture where animals are concerned – prevention is always the better option.

Poultry specialisation has been an unpopular career choice, which is probably a result of a limited amount of training and exposure; but as the importance of the meat to feeding the world population increases, both the need and demand for skilled veterinary surgeons will increase. Curriculum design will almost certainly change to reflect these needs.

FISH VETERINARY SURGEON

Pig and poultry farming are likely to increase in importance as they are some of the most efficient animals for converting the food fed to them into the muscle and fat that is desirable. Fish are another source of protein that can be exploited to supply the demand and where creatures are farmed there will be disease and the requirement for health advice. Some veterinary surgeons will give advice and carry out visits across the world and some practices will serve continents.

Many vets will treat ornamental (pet) fish but there are few vets involved in this important area of food production. The species range is large in comparison to the pig and poultry industries. Game and sea fish of many species as well as crustaceans and molluscs are farmed, and the prevention of disease is important. Again, like the pig and poultry veterinary surgeon, there is an emphasis on the biosecurity element of disease prevention using the same tools. Where there is a greater emphasis – and is an area that differs from the role of other veterinary surgeons – is the consideration of the environmental impact of the farming. This is particularly important for sensitive marine environments. Although fish will convert a large percentage of the food they are fed into bodyweight, they can also have a significant impact on marine environments. Part of the veterinary surgeon's task will be to assist fish farmers in meeting local regulations and ensuring that any impact on the local environment is minimised.

ABATTOIR VETERINARY SURGEON

To ensure that the meat produced on farms and sold to the public is safe to eat, all animals that are destined for human consumption are inspected. This inspection is overseen by a veterinary surgeon. Their role is to examine animals as they are admitted to the slaughterhouse or abattoir. In the European Union (EU), all animal species are inspected by veterinary surgeon before the meat is allowed to be sold on the open market.

The responsibilities are twofold: they are there to protect the welfare of the animal and to ensure the safety of the food produced. All the animals that enter an abattoir are inspected while alive to ensure that they have no lesions and are behaving normally. In cattle and sheep, checking for lameness is probably the most common welfare problem encountered but severe parasitism – such as sheep scab – might also be encountered. Welfare at slaughter is an important part of welfare protection and the veterinary surgeon's role is to ensure that the animals are being slaughtered in a manner that is appropriate. Humane slaughter is where the animal is rendered insensible to pain prior to death. This can be carried out by shooting with a captive bolt, passing an electrical current through the head or by making the animal breath gases that will cause unconsciousness, such as high concentrations of carbon dioxide. Once the animal is unconscious then the animal is usually bled in order to ensure death and it is recommended that this be done within a certain time. The Humane Slaughter Association is a charitable organisation that promotes the good slaughter standards and conducts research to determine what constitutes humane slaughter; UK facilities will adhere to their recommendations. Other countries will also have their own regulations.

Ensuring food safety requires that there are procedures in place to minimise contamination of the meat with potentially dangerous organisms. Food-borne diseases that can be transmitted by eating contaminated meat include E. coli O157:H7 and campylobacter, both of which cause gastroenteritis if not more severe illness. Working in an abattoir will require an understanding of the processes that stop infections causing food borne illnesses. Hazard Analysis and Critical Control Point (HACCP) is a process that is used to control risks in a manufacturing process; it was developed to produce safe food for space exploration in the 1960s. It relies on monitoring specific points in the process that will stop contamination; in abattoirs a simple example is ensuring that animals are required to be clean when they arrive at the abattoir, ensuring that minimal faeces enter the abattoir, which stops meat being tainted with bacteria from the intestine of the animal. The welfare aspects of the abattoir also have an influence on the food quality. If animals are stressed then glycogen (sugar stores) are removed as the body works to deal with stress. The processes that are required to produce edible meat require glycogen stores. If cattle are stressed and deplete these stores, this will produce dark, firm, dry beef that has poor eating and keeping qualities. Protecting welfare therefore has an economic benefit for farmers and the abattoir, as the meat from stressed animals is generally unsaleable.

As meat production fulfils more of the food requirements of the world population then the safety and the quality of the meat produced will become more important. Veterinary surgeons will be key to ensuring the safety of this food chain, from direct inspection of an individual carcase to taking the knowledge of working in a single facility and applying it to the understanding of the risk management for the entire industry. Abattoir veterinary surgeons will start early in the morning on a regular basis; as they become more involved with designing and checking the food safety monitoring programmes of a country then the time requirement will resemble an office position.

RESEARCH

There are many new treatments, concepts, diagnostic techniques and other pieces of information that are presented to society and veterinary surgeons when it comes to working with animals. Veterinary surgeons are part of the effort that goes into the understanding of the world that we live in.

There are many ways that a veterinary surgeon can become involved in research: they may be in practice and work on clinical questions relevant to their practice. Farm animal veterinary surgeons have had a long history of working with research organisations to decide on the best treatments or to monitor the amount of disease in the country where they work. In the UK, computer data mining systems are starting to be developed that will allow better data collection from practices. SAVSNET and Vet Compass are two examples of systems that allow the veterinary surgeon to contribute data during the course of their normal working day that will inform evidence-based practice.

Veterinary surgeons that wish to have a full-time career in research will often undertake further training, going on to complete a Master's degree or a PhD. This will involve further training and study, usually at a research institute or university. PhD studies are intended to be three years but may extend beyond that if the research question demands it. The question that is answered during this period as research student will depend on the natural curiosity of the student and the priorities of whatever funding organisations are relevant. Because of this require-ment to complete the research and the curiosity of the student, the hours can be very long. It can also feel a very isolated position, as there may be few who are in a position to understand the pressures that a PhD candidate is dealing with.

Once a PhD or equivalent research degree is obtained, then a research career is open to the veterinary surgeon. Associated with most research positions is a teaching role as many research staff – although not all – are appointed as lectur-ers. This will involve passing on their learning in a specific area through lectures, small group teaching, clinic teaching or any other methodology that the university employs.

PHARMACEUTICAL VETERINARY SURGEON

Pharmaceutical companies have many responsibilities associated with the sale of medicines that are used in treating animals. The companies will monitor the usage and advise where appropriate on the correct usage. Pharmacovigilance is a critical responsibility of the companies that produce them. Pharmacovigilance is the monitoring and investigation of adverse events that are potentially associ-ated with drugs supplied by the company. Veterinary surgeons are employed by companies to monitor these events and cooperate with regulatory organisations that will be interested. Where the companies are producing antibiotics then the appearance to resistance will be a priority investigation for the company, and veterinary surgeons working in the pharmaceutical industry will be part of the investigation.

Veterinary surgeons working in practice like to be involved in projects that will improve the health of animals associated with their practice. This can be facilitated by working with pharmaceutical companies, and usually the veterinary surgeons employed by the companies will be involved. The pharmaceutical company will use initiatives to raise awareness of specific conditions; although in the UK they are not permitted to market medicines directly to the public, this is not the case in all countries.

This awareness-raising of conditions is part of the education activities that pharmaceutical companies will become involved in, but companies will also be involved in the education of veterinary students. This can be by providing or sponsoring lectures on specific subjects, providing the printing of hard copies of lectures or sponsoring the purchase of equipment that will help students practice practical techniques. In the medical field there is some debate about whether this is appropriate, as pharmaceutical influence is thought to influence prescribing habits. In any case, this activity will spread new ideas throughout the veterinary and animal communities.

Employment conditions for veterinary surgeons working in the pharmaceutical industry will involve long hours and potentially international travel. As with all of the careers, the time commitment can be extensive – particularly if there are pharmacovigilance issues to deal with, which may require the veterinary surgeon to work long days and deal with the issues at weekends.

PATHOLOGIST

Veterinary pathology is a specialism that many veterinary surgeons will train for. These people will deal with animals when they are dead – examining the remains of animals to determine the cause of death. They will conduct a detailed and logical examination. This information can be used for many purposes, such as allowing farm animal veterinary surgeons to work with their clients and prevent further losses from diseases as diverse as BVD or leptospirosis. Where the animal is an individual such as a pet then the post-mortem can provide an answer that is reassuring as it will suggest, for example, that all that could be done was done.

Pathology results are sometimes used where there is a dispute; disputes can be related to the animals' diagnosis or treatment by the veterinary surgeon or they may be where a welfare problem is suggested. The results from a pathological examination may be used in a court case in order to secure a prosecution for keeping an animal in poor welfare conditions or economic redress for losses if inappropriate treatment is suggested. Where the veterinary pathologist is giving evidence then they may be acting as an expert witness that will help the court decide the facts of the case. The jurisdiction and judge ruling over each case will define the precise role played by the expert witness.

Pharmaceutical companies will also employ veterinary surgeons in a pathology role. When conducting trials in order to licence new medicines or medical devices for both the human market and the veterinary medicine market, there is a require-ment that they are tested on animals. Depending on the protocol, the subject animals may have to undergo a post-mortem examination and any that die unex-pectedly will have to be examined to determine the cause of death and help the company and the regulatory authorities decide whether the product should be marketed.

Veterinary pathologists will typically conduct the examination in a post-mortem suite. These rooms have all the equipment needed to complete the examination, including hoists, saws, knives and a host of other equipment. These are usually as part of a university, research institute or government service, and most veterinary surgeons who work as pathologists will be employed by one of these organisa-tions. Unlike many of the other career paths taken by veterinary surgeons after qualifying, driving large distances is not a major feature of this role, but long hours generally are (in common with all veterinary careers).

REFERRAL VETERINARY SURGEON

In companion animal practice, some veterinary surgeons will specialise in specific areas. They will commonly work as part of a large practice and provide an extra level of service to the owners of companion animals. Alternatively they may work as a consultant to many practices, visiting as a peripatetic (travelling) consultant and seeing clients to improve the service to clients. The veterinary surgeon will have developed a specific expertise through postgraduate training, such as:

- **Dermatology** – treating skin conditions such as allergies, parasites, tumours and hormonal issues.

- **Ophthalmology** – treating conditions affecting the eye such as glaucoma, and genetic eye defects.

- **Orthopaedic** – treating conditions affecting bones, primarily to restore movement by repairing complex fractures or treating developmental conditions of the limbs.

- **Neurology** – treating the nervous system from the spinal column to the brain itself. Repairing crushing of the spinal column, diagnosing and treating tumours in the brain as well as dealing with many other disorders.

- **Oncology** – treating cancer in patients particularly those requiring complex treatment plans with medicines that require special facilities to administer.

- **Anaesthesia and analgesia** – working to manage animals undergoing surgical operations. Veterinary surgeons who train in this specialty will manage the pain and ensure that the animal is able to breath and maintain good blood flow throughout the body, especially important when dealing with a high-risk patient.

- **Cardiology** – the heart and vascular system is an area that many veterinary surgeons will study. As animals age, the heart will start to fail in many so the ability to support these animals will become more important.

- **Soft tissue surgery** – soft tissue surgeons will work on complex cases involving the internal organs of the animal. This can be in support of other specialties, to reconstruct tissue following disease or trauma or to correct problems that are present from birth.

- **Behaviour** – many animals have behavioural problems that concern the owners and some vets will be specialists in managing these cases.

- **Diagnostic imaging** – most associated with veterinary surgeons is the ability to take X-ray images (radiographs) and these are used in surgeries and on equine yards. But there are other ways that veterinary surgeons can now get images of the deeper tissues including ultrasound, magnetic resonance imaging (MRI) and CAT scans.

- **Emergency and critical care** – companion animals are involved in accidents or are struck with sudden and life-threatening conditions; veterinary surgeons will have to deal with these regularly and some will specialise in this aspect. This has become a full-time career option, with companies being set up to provide the out-of-hours cover that veterinary surgeons are obliged to provide.

- **Dentistry** – animals need good dental care and brushing is an important part of the care of cats and dogs. Dentistry skills are needed in order to provide the extraction and cosmetic repair in some instances. A routine task is an extensive cleaning getting below the gumline. It is not possible to clean the mouth while the animal is conscious, so most dentistry is done under anaesthesia. Occasionally an individual trained in human dentistry will work on animal mouths. This is quite common with primates in zoos due to the similarity in anatomy. As they are not veterinary surgeons, these dentists are obliged to work under the supervision of a qualified vet in all locations in a similar manner to other allied professions.

ZOO VETERINARY SURGEON

There are zoos and wildlife parks all over the world and the larger ones will employ veterinary surgeons to work with their animals. These will carry out the treatment of the collection of rare and exotic animals in the zoological collection. This will involve surgical interventions, medical therapy and preventative care. The range of species that veterinary surgeons working in zoos have under their care is probably the widest of any practising vet. In a similar manner to farm animal veterinary surgeons, they will produce health plans to document and coordinate the preventative measures at the zoo or park. Again, as with other species, the environment is a crucial part of the care of animals, but environmental enrichment in zoos is important in maintaining the behaviours that wild animals are expected to exhibit. The veterinary surgeon may be involved in working with the rest of the zoo staff to design and build appropriate accommodation for the animals.

Alongside the care of the animals, the vet's responsibilities may extend to being involved in breeding programmes by measuring hormone levels, helping to move animals from place to place in order to protect the species by again helping the breeding programme of the species. This movement of animals, although helping with breeding, poses a risk of introducing a disease onto the facility. The veterinary surgeon will arrange for the testing of the animals for diseases that will put the collection at risk. These may be legally required by the government or may be required by the zoo as part of their health planning.

LABORATORY ANIMAL VETERINARY SURGEON

In the UK in 2013 there were just over four million scientific procedures involving animals, and up to 60 million animal procedures are thought to be carried out worldwide every year. Veterinary surgeons are employed in laboratories to ensure that the welfare of the animals involved in these procedures is to the highest standard.

The species that are involved in experimentations are varied – from zebra fish to cattle – as different creatures will allow different questions to be examined and the choice of animal will be important in the accuracy of the answers.

Veterinary surgeons will be involved in protecting the welfare of the animals and will decide when the animal is suffering more than is acceptable under the terms of the licence held by the experimenter. The veterinary surgeon will also be involved in developing the terms of the experimental procedure that underpins the licence. The licence will be developed with the three Rs of reduction refinement and replacement in mind, as well as considering whether the model is appropriate. Supervision of the movement of animals will also be monitored by veterinary surgeons in the UK and USA, as well as in most other countries. The veterinary surgeon will also monitor the overall health of the animals under their care. This role is very much like the role of a large animal veterinary surgeon, as the experimental animals have a task for which they are intended and diseases occurring at the same time (concurrent) – whether from unintended bacterial or viral infections – will render the results from any experiment difficult if not impossible to interpret. Welfare compromises will also have adverse effects on the results from animal experiments. Veterinary surgeons and appropriate care will ensure that the most valuable results possible are achieved.

WILDLIFE VETERINARY SURGEON

The conservation of our shared national environment is an important task and wildlife is a fundamental part of this. The biodiversity of our world and the diverse ecosystems within it require that we protect the animals. The veterinary surgeon's oath of many countries talks about animals 'under my care', and what falls into this category is a point for each individual's conscience. Wildlife should be part of the profession's responsibility and some veterinary surgeons will be involved in dealing with wildlife as a career. However, many more will get involved in this work through charities and specific projects where they will devote their time.

Rehabilitation of injured wildlife is the most evocative image of a wildlife veterinary surgeon – this could involve taking in animals that have been injured through interactions with man, natural disasters or for some other reason. This will involve all the skills that are exhibited by companion animal veterinary surgeons. As with most of veterinary medicine, preventative actions are becoming more important. Organisations will ask vets to help coordinate and deliver projects in order to protect the wildlife of a region. This could be vaccinating dogs for distemper to prevent the spread to the neighbouring tiger populations, identifying diseases that are spreading throughout endangered bird populations or training local veterinary surgeons so that the requirement for international help is reduced. Wildlife medicine is usually pictured as something that occurs in tropical places such as Africa and Asia, but wildlife preservation is required all over the world with, for example, hedgehogs in the UK and raptor rehabilitation in Europe and America. A particularly influential example of the wildlife veterinary surgeon is Gladys Kalema-Zikusoka who has worked to preserve gorillas in Uganda having identified the risk that human parasites can infect gorillas. She also was instrumental in moving animals from other parts of Africa to restock national parks following the civil war. Through her organisation Conservation Through Public Health, human health and the health of the environment are improved in parallel.

CHARITY VETERINARY SURGEON

There is always a need to provide for those owners and animals that are in need. Even in countries where there is a social care model for human healthcare, animal care is a private care model. Veterinary surgeons will provide healthcare to clients that are struggling – maybe due to loss of employment, ill-health of the owner, old age or other reasons – according to their own morals and by sourcing funds from charities, but this is unsustainable in the long term and with a large percentage of clients. In order to assist these cases, owners and animals' charities have been organised. These include the Royal/Scottish/American Society for the Prevention of Cruelty to Animals (RSPCA/SSPCA/ASPCA), the People's Dispensary for Sick Animals (PDSA) and many other small local charities. Veterinary surgeons will work for these in an enforcement role where the charity has one (the RSPCA, for example), or other veterinary surgeons will provide clinical services to the clients that meet any eligibility criteria that the charity may wish to impose. They will provide the same clinical procedures as a colleague in a more commercial environment. The charity will have limited resources and these will have to be spread throughout the recipients of the charities. This will almost certainly limit the treatment options available to the veterinary surgeon, so some antibiotics will be unavailable due to the cost. Advanced diagnostic techniques such as MRI scanning may also not be available, as the use of resources on a single animal where those resources could be used more widely is a balance that is constantly being debated and changed. This may appear to compromise the desire to provide the highest care, but such limitations can provide inspiration for the veterinary surgeon to come up with creative solutions to difficult problems.

Charities may be involved with the treatment of animal species and they work all over the world. Global charities involved in equine treatment include SPANA, Gambia Horse and Donkey Trust, Redwings, the Donkey Sanctuary, World Horse Welfare and the oldest horse-specific charity, the Horse Trust. These will provide short-term veterinary care and training to the local population in order to improve the health and welfare of horses wherever they work. Other organisations will work with cats and dogs; the PDSA in the UK will help companion animals of owners who cannot otherwise afford the treatment, while Charities such as the Worldwide Veterinary Service provide veterinary expertise to charities and shelters around the globe.

There is debate about whether those who cannot afford to keep animals should be supported in doing so, but the animals have the right to adequate treatment in order to protect their welfare. In any case, animals as companions can be an important part of a person's life and greatly improve the quality of life whether through companionship or in areas where they are work animals, providing power for agricultural and increasing food production. In either case, charities can improve human welfare by working with animals; human health is also affected by the work of charities dealing with companion animals and equines. Rabies kills tens of thousands of people each year, with dog bites being the most common way people – particularly children under the age of 15 – are infected. Vaccination of feral (abandoned) dogs combined with neutering is an approach that is used to reduce the amount (prevalence) of infected dogs and thereby the number of deaths in people.

There are many initiatives that could benefit from charitable involvement but resources are limited. The veterinary surgeon will be involved in the allocation of these resources to further the aim of the charity. The public's expectation of what can be achieved will also be important to consider, as expectations of the charity can be unrealistic.

MILITARY VETERINARY SURGEON

Animals have been part of warfare for centuries, with dogs documented as being used by the Greeks and horses associated with cavalry fighting throughout the ages. Animals have been used as weapons, as transport, to detect explosives and to deliver explosives to enemy positions. Animals have been used for communication and to maintain morale in military units. They provide security and have protected naval vessels from vermin. Marine mammals (dolphins and sea lions) have been trained to protect seaborne forces from mines and underwater incursion. Intelligence-gathering and chemical weapons detection have also been attempted with varying degrees of success.

Dogs and horses have probably been the most commonly used animals in war but pigeons, elephants, camels, oxen, sea lions and dolphins have all been used. Other animals have been suggested down the ages but it is uncertain whether they were actually used in battle. Although humans started using animals in warfare almost as soon as warfare started, the practice continues to this day with dogs used for security, attack and explosive detection. The horse has been used as a way to transport men into battle and even in modern conflicts the horse has been reported as carrying Special Forces soldiers into remote terrain. The Indian army maintains the 61st cavalry that is the world's largest non-ceremonial horse regiment. China is believed to use horse-mounted troops in small numbers to patrol its land borders.

The majority of countries that field military forces will have a veterinary force – termed variously a corps, service, centre or directorate – to provide for the animals in the army. The members of these units will be full-time military personnel or operate in a part-time (reserve) capacity. The animals in any army have to perform to their best or the lives of serving personnel will be endangered. The veterinary services of any country will ensure that animals are cared for and treated with the best options available. The role of the army veterinary surgeon will not stop at treating the animals owned by the military force, whether those forces are air, land or sea. The role depends on the national resources designated to the corps or services but commonly involves public health issues as qualified veterinary surgeons have prior training in this discipline, along with advising command elements on the control of zoonotic diseases.

Military forces are also involved in emergency relief, post-conflict rebuilding and in non-traditional conflicts such as the operations in Afghanistan. Working with the local communities to rebuild communities, farms and provide the equine power is a vital role and contributes to the national interest of the county of origin.

The veterinary services of the armed forces work in dangerous places alongside fellow professionals to bring aid to the people and animals of countries where strife has made life difficult. Veterinary surgeons have lost their lives in war. Lieutenant Vincent Fox was the first member of the RCVS to be killed when he died in World War I, while Lieutenant Colonel Daniel Holland was killed in 2006 while performing his duties as a veterinary surgeon for the US Army in Iraq. Their work and the work of the animal handlers that have also fallen (such as Lance Corporal Liam Iasker and Lance Corporal Kenneth Rowe) will be remembered and will contribute to the safety and security of all the countries involved. It is always the hope that no more sacrifice is required.

LOCUM VETERINARY SURGEON

A final category of career that many veterinary surgeons undertake is that of a locum veterinary surgeon. Locum veterinary surgeons will provide holiday cover, maternity cover and sick cover for veterinary practices in the UK, Australia and New Zealand. In other countries, the service is referred to as relief cover.

Veterinary surgeons who work as locums will move from practice to practice allowing other veterinary surgeons to have holidays or go on maternity leave. Locums will replace sick veterinary surgeons in order to allow the level of service to be maintained by a practice.

This is a popular way of working, as it allows a great deal of flexibility in when the veterinary surgeon works – although when no work is available, the veterinary surgeon will have no income. If there is an ambition to own a practice, then this will potentially compromise the ability to pursue this.

To carry out the responsibilities of a locum veterinary surgeon requires some experience, as the employing practice will require that the locum will have adequate experience to drop into a position and carry out at least the routine tasks effectively and efficiently. This applies whether the locum works in companion, equine, farm or any other aspect of the veterinary industry. It is probably wise to have a few years' experience of the particular branch of veterinary medicine that the locum position involves before getting involved.

VETERINARY CAREERS

When most people describe a veterinary surgeon they will probably talk about a person wearing a white coat or scrubs and a stethoscope, examining and treating an animal or operating to cure a problem. They may talk about a person wearing wellington boots standing behind a cow or wearing a protective coverall and watching a horse. The role of a veterinary surgeon is much wider than this. Veterinary surgeons are involved in research that can be critical in protecting human health directly and indirectly. All food of animal origin in Europe, the USA and Australia is inspected by veterinary surgeons. Other veterinary surgeons will develop the legislative framework that protects the health and welfare of farmed, companion and wild animals. The veterinary surgeons may only look at one aspect of animal health or one species. They can support the military and strategic objectives of their country through military service. Veterinary surgeons can work in government offices, clinics, research labs and many other environments. The careers in this chapter are those that a veterinary surgeon may choose if they qualify today, but changes in society and the profession may add or remove some of these and will almost certainly change the numbers of veterinary surgeons employed in these roles.

What all these career options have in common is that they have a high degree of professional responsibility and associated stress. The hours are long and the work is frequently routine and repetitive, although there is also a significant amount of intellectual challenge. Balancing these two facets can be a challenge for many veterinary surgeons.

The veterinary degree is a good science degree and can be used in many careers. These may not be in the veterinary field and even if after all of the training or a period of experience in the profession you decide that a change of direction is required, then many other positions can be taken on – from working in finance to becoming a manager in a multinational company.

7

VETS AND ECONOMICS

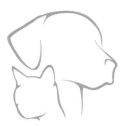

All of veterinary medicine is a business: studying to become a veterinary surgeon requires paying to study; treating an animal requires paying for advice and drugs. The ability to carry out the tasks of diagnosing and treating animals requires an extensive support network and this will all come with an economic cost. This ranges from cleaners to the research required to develop new treatments to manage and cure diseases. When veterinary surgeons work on disease control at national levels then the economics of whole countries may become important. At all levels there is an economic consideration to veterinary medicine.

THE COST OF STUDYING

Student fees

To provide training and the education required for the production of a highly skilled professional costs money. Universities require a large lecturing staff in disciplines from physiology to law and many others. These require support staff that are skilled in the appropriate techniques relevant to the lecturing staff. There will be significant investment in educational materials such as printed notes, online learning materials and cadavers for anatomy lessons. These lessons will require a suitable building in which they can be carried out. This can be the traditional lecture hall, laboratory, dissecting room or smaller seminar rooms. These require heating, electricity, computer and internet capabilities, maintenance and all after they have first been built! These are in common with any other course, but veterinary schools also have to invest in clinics that can attract the cases that will provide a valuable educational experience. This means providing high-class facilities for companion animal, equine and farm animal care and there are a number of models that are used to deliver this for the student body. Studies require libraries with staff and textbooks as well as space to work.

There is also the social aspect of studying, as it is important that the aspiring veterinary student population has a social life as well. This can include sports centres and cafeterias as well as other meeting places.

All of this has to be paid for and a large proportion will be through student fees. In the UK the maximum a student born in the country (a home student) will pay is £9,000 per year in tuition fees. These are the fees paid to the university that cover the teaching costs of the student. On top of these will be the living costs associated with university life. For international students the fees are between £20,000 and £36,000. Fees are likely to change depending on application date, government policy for supporting higher education and university requirements.

Fees in the USA follow a similar structure, with students from within the state having lower fees than those from outside the state. Where a state has no veterinary college within its boundaries, they may establish an agreement where its residents can pay as if they are studying in-state. The relevant states are covered by the Western Interstate Commission for Higher Education (WICHE). The costs in 2014 for veterinary education ranged from $15,377 per year to $62,084, a

TABLE 7.1 Indicative fees for veterinary schools in the UK.

University	UK student fees	International fees
University of Bristol	£9,000	£33,900.00
University of Cambridge	£9,000	£36,459.00
University of Edinburgh	£9,000	£29,000.00
University of Glasgow	£9,000 (for Scottish students)	£25,500.00
University of Liverpool	£9,000	£29,950.00
University of Nottingham	£9,000	£26,970.00
Royal Veterinary College	£9,000	£25,750.00
University of Surrey	£9,000	£15,615.00

more detailed breakdown is given in Table 7.2. These figures are provided as an indication of the financial implications of choosing to study veterinary medicine. The costs of college tuition are likely to change over time and are most likely to increase but before choosing a college you should confirm the costs with your college of choice.

TABLE 7.2 Indicative fees for veterinary schools in the United States of America.

Auburn University	$17,440.00	$17,440.00	$41,172.00
University of California – Davis	$33,091.00	$45,336.00	$45,336.00
Colorado State University	$25,242.00	$25,242.00	$53,218.00
Cornell University	$29,400.00	—	$44,250.00
University of Florida	$28,100.00	—	$45,500.00
University of Georgia	$17,078.00	$25,800.00	$42,878.00
University of Illinois	$28,446.00	—	$44,910.00
Iowa State University	$19,581.00	varies by contract	$41,390.00
Kansas State University	$22,403.60	—	$48,897.20
Louisiana State University	$19,552.00	$19,552.00	$45,352.00
Michigan State University	$26,016.00	—	$52,206.00
University of Minnesota	$32,456.00	—	$56,210.00
Mississippi State University	$18,011.00	$18,011.00	$43,011.00
University of Missouri	$20,092.00	—	$49,398.00

University			
North Carolina State University	$15,377.56	—	$38,140.56
Ohio State University	$28,620.00	—	$62,084.00 (can apply for residency after first year)
Oklahoma State University	$16,640.00	—	$36,900.00
Oregon State University	$21,386.00	$21,386.00	$40,690.00
University of Pennsylvania	$37,304.00	—	$46,993.00
Purdue University	$19,326.00	—	$44,154.00
University of Tennessee	$22,616.00	—	$49,142.00
Texas A&M University	$20,478.00	—	$31,278.00
Tufts University	$41,062.00	—	$44,346.00
Tuskegee University	$10,860.00 per semester ($21,720 per year)	—	$18,135.00 per semester ($36,270 per year)
Virginia- Maryland Regional	$21,434.00	—	$46,366.00
Washington State University	$22,378.00	$21,830.0	$53,422.00
Western University of Health Sciences	$47,055.00	—	$47,055.00
University of Wisconsin	$19,036.24	—	$25,880.56

TABLE 7.3 Indicative fees for schools in other regions. This is not a complete list of all possible colleges.

University	Home student fees	International fees
CEU Cardenal Herrera University	€14,600.00	€14,600.00
University of Calgary	$5,432.10	Not available
University College Dublin	€19,500.00	€33,500.00
University of Forestry - Sofia	€5,000.00	€5,000.00
University of Guelph	$C 8,609.50	$C 53,554.58
Massey University	$NZ10,826.80	Year 1 $NZ40,456.00– to $NZ54,600.00 Years 2–5 $NZ54,600.00
University of Melbourne	AU$10,085.00	AU$54,688.00
National Autonomous University of Mexico	$2,000 USD	$2,000 USD

TABLE 7.3 continued

University	Home student fees	International fees
Université de Montréal	$CAN 3251.70	$CAN 8787. 15
Murdoch University	AU$46,000.00	AU$46,000.00
University of Prince Edward Island (AVC)	C$12,308.00	C$54,759.00
University of Queensland	AU$9,517.00	AU$54,080.00
Ross University	N/A	$17,725.00 to $22,250.00 per semester
University of Saskatchewan	C$9,051.95	C$9,051.95
St. George's University	Years 1–3 $33,368.00 Year 4 $59,202.00	Years 1–3 $33,368.00 Year 4 $59,202.00
Trakia University	€3,300.00	€5,000.00
University of Sydney	AU$9,021.00	AU$37,500.00
Utrecht University	€1,951.00	€18,500.00

COST OF LIVING AT UNIVERSITY

The cost of tuition is only part of the costs associated with university education. There needs to be someplace to live and the variation on this will depend on the location, whether it is university-managed or private, the number of flatmates and the standard required. Food and clothing – some of which will be protective clothing required for the course such as lab coats, boots, waterproof trousers and jackets, protective coveralls – also need to be budgeted for.

For many students the holidays between semesters or terms are an ideal opportunity to (among other activities) work and build up a financial reserve. However, veterinary students are expected to complete extra-mural studies (EMS) of many forms in the holiday periods. Although this type of expectation is not unique to veterinary medicine students, the obligation will reduce or eliminate the opportunity to work and produce the financial cushion that would be so helpful during term-time.

PAYING FOR TRAINING

All of the costs associated with training a veterinary surgeon will have to be paid for. Some will be paid for by government sponsorship, while some will be paid by the student themselves either through loans from government programmes or other commercial organisations.

The UK administers the payment of loans for fees and living costs (maintenance loans) through the student loans company. Repayment will be collected alongside taxes through the UK's PAYE system. The rate of interest of repayment is linked to the retail price index (a measure of inflation in the economy) or the base rate of a specific set of banks. Maximum amounts are available for maintenance depending on means testing and the student's specific situation. Australia has a similar system of loans, grants and support for its students.

The situation in the USA is very similar with government (federal) loans and private loans available to the student. Unlike in the UK, the student will be expected to fund the whole of tuition fees (in the UK the government will at least partially cover tuition).

Most students therefore will have a debt upon graduation that will have to be repaid and the amount will depend on the method used to pay for tuition and living costs while at university. This will probably be a bigger debt in those who have completed their veterinary training by paying for it as a second degree as is normal among American students but increasingly common for other students. This debt will have a large influence on employment choices after graduation, as repayments will have to be made.

THE EXPECTED SALARY

Veterinary surgeons are thought to be well paid and able to afford good holidays, cars and homes. This is frequently mentioned when the costs of veterinary care are discussed, with the salary thought to be the main reason that the costs of treatment are so high. It is commonly thought and commented upon that veterinary surgeons attract high salaries – however, this needs to be put in the context of training levels and the purchasing power of any profession.

Salaries in the UK

UK vets are regularly surveyed by a number of organisations including the Society of Practising Veterinary Surgeons (SPVS) and the Royal College of Veterinary Surgeons (RCVS). These surveys (like all such surveys) are dependent on the data that is collected and the accuracy of the respondents in their answers but they do give an indication of the salary that can be expected. In 2011 the average (mean) salary for a vet was £29,622 and by 2014 this had increased to £31,150 according to a survey carried out by the RCVS. A more recent survey by the SPVS showed that companion animal veterinary surgeons were paid an average of £41,148, which was a slight increase (0.4 per cent) on the previous survey. Equine veterinary surgeons had an average salary of £43,000. Mixed practice – such as was practiced by James Herriot – now attracts an average salary of £41,176, while those concerned purely with food animal production have an average salary of £44,142. All of these categories of veterinary surgeons have increased in salary over the past few years but two categories that have decreased are those in industry and those in academia and research, whose salaries have apparently decreased in response to the financial crisis and a downturn in spending. Veterinary surgeons working for the pharmaceutical companies have also suffered from the downturn in spending by both government and public with average salaries of £59,106.

In most industries due to historical reasons there is a difference between the amount that women members of the profession get paid in comparison to the male members. This was about a 10 per cent difference in 2014. Hopefully this will come down in the next few years.

Not many years ago a vet's salary package would have included a house, car and mobile phone, but tax regulations have made it more attractive to remove all of these benefits for a purely cash-based salary package.

Comparison with other jobs

The salaries of other positions in the UK are surveyed by the Office for National Statistics (ONS). The table below indicates the mean salary of a selection of jobs that we can use to place the salary in context. Like all summaries of a complex situation a single figure can be misleading. Individual salaries may be very different from those presented here due to the location that the person is working, the organisation and, sadly, the gender.

TABLE 7.4 Average salaries in the UK, 2014

Job title	Average salary
Chief executives and senior officials	£117,700.00
Human resource managers and directors	£54,120.00
Senior officers in protective services	£55,162.00
Senior police officers	£58,727.00
Senior officers in fire, ambulance, prison and related services	£49,684.00
Health services and public health managers and directors	£49,015.00
Science, research, engineering and technology professionals	£41,429.00
Natural and social science professionals	£38,202.00
Chemical scientists	£35,492.00
Civil engineers	£38,236.00
Mechanical engineers	£44,176.00
Electrical engineers	£44,439.00
Electronics engineers	£36,751.00
Health professionals	£54,329.00
Medical practitioners	£70,648.00
Psychologists	£34,174.00
Pharmacists	£36,739.00
Ophthalmic opticians	£30,959.00
Dental practitioners	£53,567.00
Medical radiographers	£31,505.00
Podiatrists	£28,125.00
Records clerks and assistants	£19,146.00
Pensions and insurance clerks and assistants	£22,694.00
Stock control clerks and assistants	£20,891.00
Transport and distribution clerks and assistants	£23,583.00
Library clerks and assistants	£12,190.00

Due to the sampling differences between the different groups who look at the earning potential of the veterinary profession, the stated average salary can differ – for the ONS the average salary for a veterinary surgeon is estimated to be £32,374.00 which is comparable with other medical professions such as ophthalmologists but less than the doctors or dentists. Whether this appropriate remuneration is a complex question but assuming that this will not change, then the prospective veterinary surgeon should expect to receive these amounts and should expect to have a lifestyle that such a salary can support.

SALARIES IN THE USA

Veterinary associations in the USA also survey their members. For those working in America the median salary for veterinary surgeons that work with a limited species mix is $100,000. Working in a mixed practice appears to reduce the salary. This may reflect the location of these veterinary surgeons. Salaries for those in corporate or government areas are slightly higher, with the median being $124,000.

The bureau of labour statistics supplies data similar to that provided by the ONS in the UK. The average salary of a veterinary surgeon is certainly reasonable but it must be remembered that debts may be higher.

TABLE 7.5 Average salaries in the US, 2014

Job description	Average salary
Top executives	$121,010.00
Chief executives	$178,400.00
General and operations managers	$116,090.00
Transportation, storage, and distribution managers	$91,220.00
Compensation and benefits managers	$112,040.00
Human resources managers	$111,180.00
Training and development managers	$107,770.00
Farmers, ranchers, and other agricultural managers	$73,210.00
Aerospace engineering and operations technicians	$62,540.00
Civil engineering technicians	$49,380.00
Electrical and electronics engineering technicians	$58,770.00
Electro-mechanical technicians	$54,160.00
Environmental engineering technicians	$49,180.00
Industrial engineering technicians	$54,170.00
Agricultural and food scientists	$64,830.00
Animal scientists	$72,930.00
Food scientists and technologists	$65,340.00
Soil and plant scientists	$62,830.00

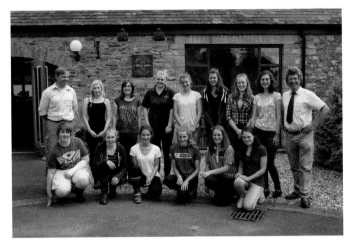

Prospective veterinary students and lecturers starting a course to gain insight into the veterinary profession.

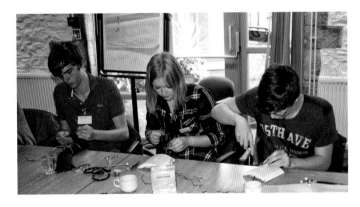

Students at a pre-vet course getting their first taste of surgery on simulator kits.

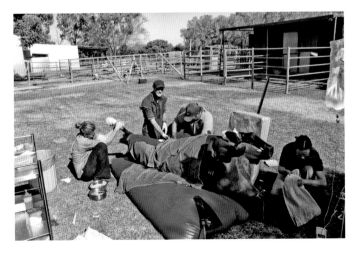

Veterinary EMS can lead to seeing many different experiences such as equine castration in the Australian sun.

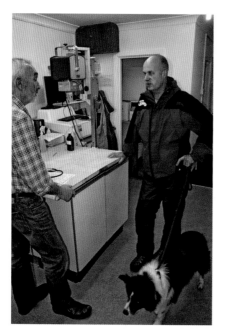

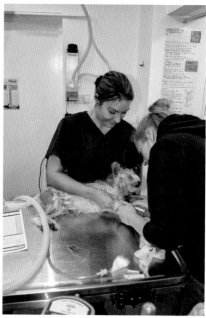

A veterinary surgeon discussing an animal's condition – good client communication will aid in getting the best information to help the diagnosis.

Veterinary surgeon and veterinary nurse working together to anaesthetise a dog.

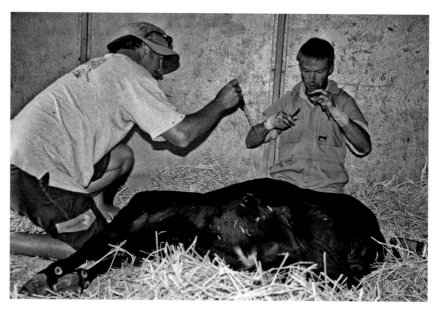

The author working on an animal to treat a deep-seated abscess. Not all surgical operations will be carried out in a sterile operating theatre.

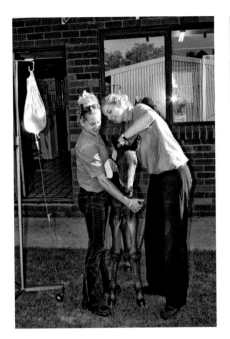

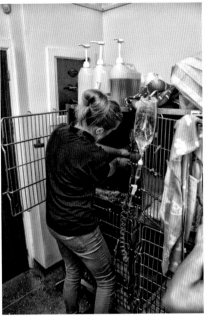

Veterinary nurses working with a sick foal. The continuous care that nurses can give can be crucial to the success of treatment.

A veterinary surgeon giving intravenous fluid therapy (IVFT) for acute renal failure (ARF). The potential list of acronyms in the veterinary field is bewildering.

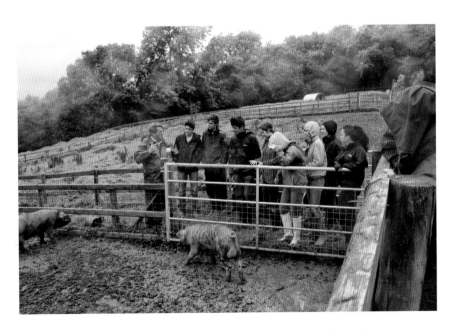

Students interested in applying to a veterinary medicine course getting a farmer's point of view on the issues relevant to farming pigs.

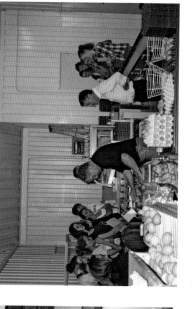

Prospective applicants to the veterinary course learning about the poultry industry and a vet's role in it.

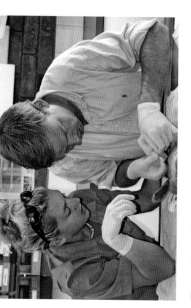

The author – who is a MRCVS, has a BVM&S and is a member of the BVA – working with a nurse.

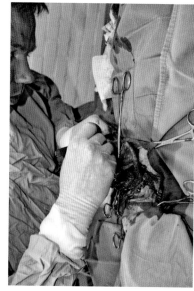

An amputation being carried out on a cat. How much would this operation cost if carried out on a human?

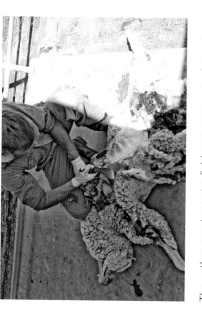

The author carrying out a field post-mortem to determine the cause of illness in a group of Australian sheep.

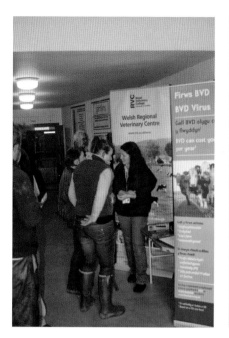

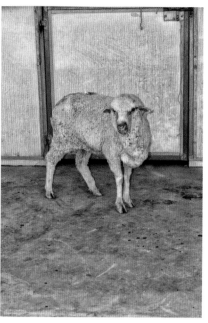

A veterinary surgeon trying to promote bovine viral diarrhoea (BVD) at a national level. This disease, if investment is made, will have a benefit to the entire farming community.

The sheep pictured is ill and potentially could be treated but the outcome is uncertain. An alternative is to euthanase the sheep and carry out a post mortem to decide what can be done to improve the growth rate of the rest of the flock. Is this ethical?

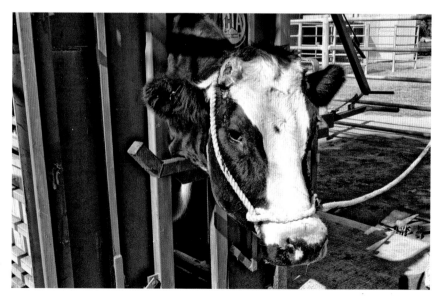

Dehorning a cow late in life to make it safer for the owner. The animal will get no benefit from this so is it ethical?

Cattle are frequently kept in sheds – is this a welfare-friendly shed for cattle?

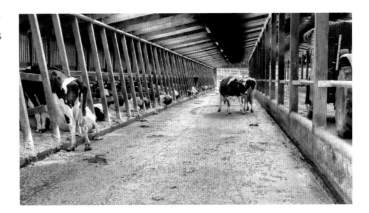

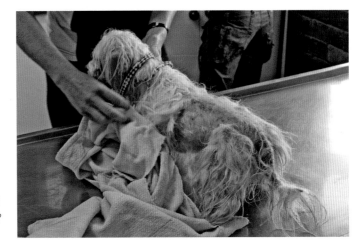

Should this animal have been presented for treatment earlier? Is it suffering?

Government veterinary surgeons from across Europe training to deal with a disease outbreak. This may require interventions at farm, regional, national and international levels. This will require interaction with politicians.

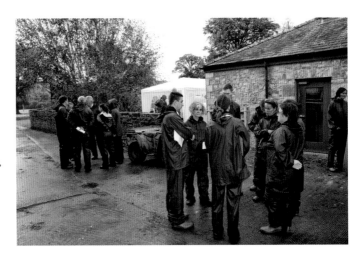

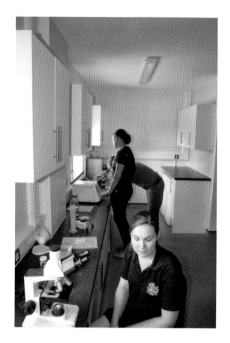

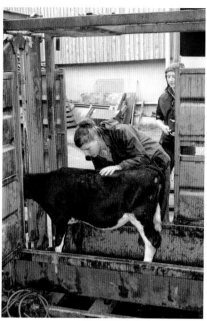

Students using microscopes in a basic laboratory setting and carrying out research on faecal samples from sheep.

Practising clinical examination on a calf.

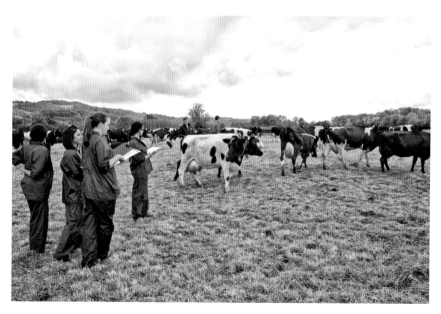

Veterinary students collecting on-farm data. Not all research is carried out in a laboratory. Epidemiology may require going out to farms and clinics and recording the number of cases seen.

Prospective students examining samples under a microscope as they learn about anthelmintic resistance issues on a sheep farm.

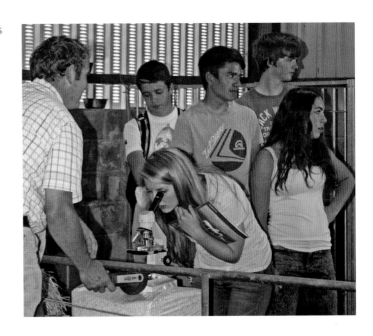

A veterinary surgeon taking a blood sample to determine the level of immunity in the calf. This will aid the vet in giving appropriate preventative advice.

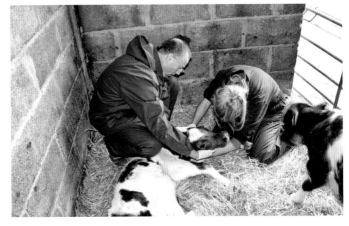

Discussing the views of a sheep farmer and learning how all the decisions have to be applied on a farm owned by a farmer.

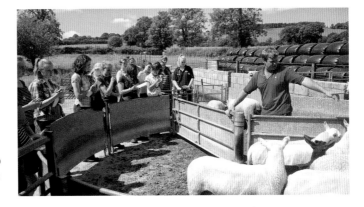

Job description	Average salary
Biological scientists	$77,630.00
Biochemists and biophysicists	$91,640.00
Parts salespersons	$32,290.00
Retail salespersons	$25,370.00
Sales representatives, services	$68,680.00
Advertising sales agents	$57,440.00
Insurance sales agents	$63,610.00
Farmworkers and labourers, crop, nursery, and greenhouse	$20,080.00
Farmworkers, farm, ranch, and aquacultural animals	$24,760.00
Agricultural workers, all other	$29,170.00
Electricians	$53,560.00
Glaziers	$42,560.00

SALARIES IN OTHER PARTS OF THE WORLD

The salary of veterinary surgeons in Australia starts at $45,000 and according to the local veterinary association, for most veterinary surgeons they will reach the top of their earning potential after five years at $75,000. Some veterinary surgeons will develop specialisms and develop the ability to sell their skills for more income.

In New Zealand, the median salary for vets according to the department of primary industries is $70,000. This may reflect a need for veterinary surgeons in New Zealand.

TABLE 7.6 Veterinary salaries worldwide, 2014

Country	Guideline salary (local currency)
UK	£31,000 (average)
USA	$100,00 (average)
Canada	$81,000 (average)
Australia	$45,000 to $75,000 (starting to maximum)
New Zealand	$70,000 (average)
South Africa	R313,000 (average)
Singapore	$50,000 (average)
Finland	€30,000 starting salary
Various European countries	€30,00 to €140,000

The salaries in Table 7.6 are all expressed in the currency local to the veterinary surgeon working in that country. It is important to remember the cost of living in each place may be very different – the cost of food, accommodation and things such as cinema tickets will influence the overall attractiveness of the salary.

Some veterinary surgeons will not work for a salary but will set up on their own, and this model is almost exclusively used in Spain, Portugal and Belgium. The profit and hence the salary depends on the efficiency and costs involved in running a business.

THE COST OF TREATING ANIMALS

Veterinary surgeons charge clients in order to treat their animals and all the work that goes into supporting this must be charged to someone. This includes everything from the bill for cleaning the practice to paying for the latest diagnostic equipment and it all has to contribute – even the additional training that is required by the veterinary surgeon. All clients will be given a bill at the end of a treatment whether that is a single examination or a long and complex therapy. This may be paid all at once or the owner (particularly with farms) may pay at the end of a fixed time (for example, monthly).

What goes into a veterinary bill?

Companion animal owners will be presented with a bill at the end of the consult but what goes into the total? There are many components and it is important to carefully consider all the influences. A very low bill may not represent the best value for owner and pet.

Advice

A veterinary surgeon will examine the animal, ask history and give advice based on the examination. This requires time, which must be accounted for and the price charged will depend on a number of factors, such as the location of the practice – as some places have a higher cost to set up as a veterinary practice. Not least, the amount of training that the veterinary surgeons undertake may be reflected in the cost to get their advice. Highly qualified veterinary surgeons with additional qualifications will in all likelihood charge a higher price for their advice, which – while not infallible – is more likely to give a suitable outcome. The hourly rate will vary from area to area and country to country. As an example, £120 per hour is a good indication of the rates that are typically charged in the UK but may be much higher.

Diagnostic tests

It may be required to conduct more detailed investigations in order to confirm or define more accurately what the diagnosis actually is. This will make the treatment plan more accurate but they come at a financial cost. Once again each practice will charge its clients differently for each diagnostic test. Blood tests in the UK can vary from £45 to £180 depending on exactly what is being tested for. In-house tests for liver enzymes or kidney enzymes may be relatively cheap. More esoteric tests to identify rare or unusual diseases may be sent off to commercial laboratories and consequently may be more expensive. X-rays may well cost £200 when the anaesthesia costs are considered. Any test will come with a cost and this cost includes the technical skill required to get the correct sample required in order to get a meaningful result, the skill to run the test, the investment in the equipment to run the test and the ability to correctly interpret the test.

Medications

The cost of medicines charged as a result of the diagnosis can be extremely variable. If the medicine is one that has been used for a long time and no single company manufactures it then it may be relatively cheap; for example, penicillin has been used for many years and can be manufactured by any authorized manufacturer and this should push prices down. A specific manufacturer may have developed other drugs; that company will be looking to recoup the investment in this drug as well as many others that failed. The manufacturing process itself may be extremely complex and require expensive starting materials, equipment and be energy-intensive. The medicine needs to be marketed to the owners and vets in order to ensure that all the options are available for treating a particular condition. Legislative costs will also have to be paid; these include safety and efficacy testing, quality control at manufacture and monitoring for side-effects once marketed. All of the costs are built into the price of the medicine that is ultimately paid by the owner.

Consumables

The term 'consumables' refers to materials that are used in veterinary practice such as syringes, needles, bandages, catheters, bungs and many other things. These have to be paid for and, once again, these costs have to be passed on to the owner.

Fees in ambulatory practice

Obviously not all veterinary surgeons work in a practice and these individuals will have to travel to the animals, whether that is on a farm, equine yard, poultry unit or somewhere else. This means that the veterinary surgeon will have to travel to the animals in order to work with them; usually this occurs by road and the veterinary surgeon will have less chargeable time per day as they will spend time travelling. In order to offset this, there may be a visit fee, which is frequently charged on the distance travelled, and once the vet has started work they may charge on either time spent or on the nature of the task being carried out.

UK fees for farm animal veterinary surgeons are similar to those for companion animal practice with chargeable time varying from £120–180 per hour as a guide but as with all of these issues some may (justifiably) charge outside this range. Equine veterinary chargeable time is costed at similar rates. The other components of a bill are the same as for those companion animals.

Comparison to human treatment costs

That veterinary surgeons are expensive is a comment that is frequently heard in the media, on internet forums and when discussing the ambition to become a veterinary surgeon. There are many reasons why the costs of veterinary medicine are high from the cost of education (both undergraduate and postgraduate training such as continuing professional development) to the cost of medications. In countries where the medical treatment of people is not paid at the point of need but through a taxpayer-funded system – such as in the UK – there is a lack of understanding of the costs of human healthcare in order to provide a useful comparison.

As examples the table below gives indicative costs for human operations. The costs are from http//privatehealth.co.uk.

TABLE 7.7 Comparison to human treatment costs

Surgical procedure	Average human cost	Indication of veterinary costs	Comment
Radiograph (X-ray)	£200	£150–250	People do not require sedation or anaesthesia.
Cruciate ligament repair	£6294	£3295	Vet price from a referral centre.
Hysterectomy	£6,044	£75–250	Neutering female dogs or cats is the equivalent procedure.
MRI scan	£490	£1213	People do not require sedation or anaesthesia. Price from university website.
Hip replacement	£10,340	£4,500	

These examples are from the UK for procedures requiring hospitalisation but the same comments are seen when searching the topic from all corners of the world and the same sort of comparisons are made. Veterinary medicine compares favourably with human medicine in terms of costs when considering the companion animal sector. Food production medicine has only a limited number of procedures that could conceivably be compared to human medicines. A full medical examination of 30 minutes may cost £130 or more and caesarean section in people may cost £3,790 or more. Where food animal production differs is that the actual cost is probably not as important as the ability to demonstrate that the investment in veterinary services is cost-effective.

Equine services are likely to be more expensive than the equivalent companion animal services even if it is purely due to the generally increased size of the animals. The economic return of this investment may be important to owners who are racing animals and expect them to win prize money.

Insurance

Although the cost of veterinary medicine is in fact reasonable in comparison to the costs associated with human medicine it can be expensive to treat animals. The costs have been outlined already and as the techniques become more advanced they will probably become more expensive.

To control the cost to the owner, many companies offer pet insurance. This will cover the pet if it becomes ill or is injured. It is possible that the owner can save money on a monthly basis but if the animal needs treatment within the first few months then the cost may exceed the accumulated savings. This will not be the case where pet insurance is taken out (although the terms and conditions need to be checked).

Many veterinary surgeons will ask the owner if they have insurance during a consultation. This may be one of the first questions that the owner is asked. This is sometimes seen as the veterinary surgeon looking for the chance to increase the final bill, but in reality most vets will be using this information to decide which of the options available are most suitable. This is a difficult balancing act as some clients will be insulted if it is assumed that they cannot afford the best treatment option for their animal, while others may be embarrassed that they cannot do so. Other clients will not wish to pay large amounts even if cost is not a barrier. Pet insurance allows the veterinary surgeon to have fewer issues with the costs of treatment.

This does not mean that any test or treatment can be applied to the case, the professional responsibility of the veterinary surgeon to carry out only those tests and treatments that are believed to be of benefit to the animals under the veterinary surgeons care still applies.

RUNNING A PRACTICE

No veterinary surgeon works as an isolated entity. There are many elements that are required within the practice environment that are involved in the efficient running of a practice.

What is required?

Staff

There are a number of staff involved in the running of a practice – not all of which are in a position to earn fees as part of their day-to-day job. Staff that are required include cleaners, accountants, managers and nurses. Nurses will potentially (depending on the practice) have the opportunity to earn fees from the practice but the other staff members will not. These staff are vital to the smooth and efficient running of the practice and they have to be paid from the fees that are earned by the practice.

Equipment

Veterinary equipment is expensive to purchase, maintain and run. Diagnostic tools that will be in a veterinary practice range from the simple pen torches that will cost a few pounds or less to MRI scanners that will cost in the millions. Other tools that you will find at a veterinary practice include stethoscopes, which can cost from a few pounds to many hundreds depending on the quality and specification of the equipment.

TABLE 7.8 The cost of veterinary equipment

Equipment	Guideline price	Use/comment
Refractometer	£10–320	Examining the concentration in bodily fluids.
Blood glucose monitor	£20–500	Monitoring diabetes.
Ophthalmoscope	£20–2,000	Indirect ophthalmoscopes are the more expensive types.
Ultrasound scanner	£2,000+	Very variable costs.
Centrifuge	£300–2,000	Spinning down fluids to aid testing.

There are many other items that are required including blood analysers, fluid pumps, scissors and surgical equipment, autoclaves and computers, as well as the required software. This all can be very expensive to buy and run, and in some cases the veterinary practice cannot fulfil its primary function without many of them. For example, surgery would be difficult without autoclaves and surgical equipment, it might be impossible to diagnose and plan the treatment of some surgical conditions without some of the imaging equipment.

Buildings

Veterinary surgeons require someplace to work; this can be a simple room where a farm animal vet can sit and work on accounts, reports and other paperwork, or it may be expanded to allow laboratory testing to be done by the veterinary surgeon himself (in-house). Companion animal vets will require consultation rooms and surgical areas and the preparation rooms associated with these. In addition there will be animal accommodation suitable for all of the species that the veterinary surgeons routinely expect to treat. As the more obvious requirements appear (consulting rooms and surgical suites), then more support rooms are required such as offices for support staff, medicine and equipment storage and cleaning stores. The costs of these can range from £100,000 to many millions depending on the specification and requirements of the practice. Alongside the specification, wherever the practice is built will also have an influence on the overall cost of the building and this applies worldwide.

The apparent expense of a building may be a barrier to some clients, as they will perceive that the majority of the bills are to pay for the buildings. Successful practices that provide a good service will be able to afford to invest in the infrastructure of the business and provide an even better service. Although a guide, the building cannot tell the client all they need to know about the level of veterinary service available.

CHARITY VETERINARY MEDICINE

Civilized society, it has been suggested, is judged by the protection that it gives to its weaker members such as children, the disabled and animals. Where animals are in situations that require treatment but there are no resources available, the animal charities have been set up to cover this gap.

Veterinary medicine is a business; the medicines, staff, equipment and infrastructure all cost money and for each practice there will be a minimum amount of money that is required to be brought in each week. This means that there will almost always be a number of animals whose owners will not be able to afford the fees levied by the practice. To fill this void, many charities have arisen such as the People's Dispensary for Sick Animals (PDSA) in the UK, the American Society for Prevention of Cruelty to Animals (ASPCA) or the Australian Animal Rescue. These will provide care to animals depending on the rules that they are operating under, as set by the trustees of the charity. This requires professionals in all the same roles as for any other veterinary practice.

Right to appropriate treatment

Animals presented to the veterinary surgeon working for a charity require all the consideration that any other animal presented would get. This might be defined as the best treatment available or it might be another option. As an example, osteosarcoma in the dog is a serious cancer condition of the leg and can be treated by amputation (removal) of the affected limb, which is a relatively low-cost option when compared with a procedure to spare the limb and allow the animal to move normally.

Appropriate use of charitable resources

Each charity will have a limited amount of resources to achieve its aims – whatever these are – and treating animals with the most up-to-date and expensive treatments will deplete these resources and reduce the number of animals that are able to be treated overall. Veterinary surgeons working in this environment will have this balancing act in their minds when working in this environment. It will manifest in using generic medications where possible. This can be difficult in that it may be that the veterinary surgeon treating the animal may feel that the branded version that is more expensive will (for good reasons) be a better option and they will have to consider the overall benefit to the animal population.

More importantly where resources are limited then prevention advice to minimise the occurrence of disease is critical.

Where charities are involved in farm animal care, treatment may be possible but euthanasing a small amount of the animals may allow a better use of resources to get an overall better outcome for all animals and this may be appropriate for companion animal charities as well. In disaster relief, triage of very sick or injured animals may also allow a better overall outcome for the animals involved. This is an extremely difficult and sensitive area for consideration.

Public responsibility

The existence of charity is a public good but does not take away the responsibility of the owners to provide for their animals. This includes adequate food of a suitable nature and accommodation where the animal can exhibit its natural behaviour. There should also be access to rapid and appropriate treatment in order to minimise the suffering the animal has to endure.

THE COST BENEFIT FOR PRODUCTION ANIMALS

For the veterinary surgeon working with production animals that are intended to produce food that can be sold, in addition to the success of treatment the expense of any treatment must be balanced against the expected return for that animal. Clearly this can be difficult to achieve in all cases and many diseases that the farm animal veterinary surgeon will deal with the population as a whole will be affected by, and the animal that is presented as sick will be the tip of the iceberg. This leads to the current thinking that prevention is better than cure and most if not all veterinary surgeons will look to work with farming clients in order to prevent disease and improve the welfare of the animals on the farm. In order to demonstrate that preventative interventions provide a benefit to the farmer, complex economic models are developed to show how diseases spread. These might look at the costs of underlying metabolic diseases such as ketosis and the costs of treatment options that might be employed from changing the management of their animals to medicating with intraruminal boli, changing the management of calves to eliminate respiratory disease with or without vaccines.

COST BENEFIT AT A NATIONAL LEVEL

Veterinary surgeons are involved in working with national-level programmes, whether these are aimed at the farm industry (which is probably the most common) or any of the other species. Frequently these are evaluated on a cost–benefit ratio as the government that supplies the money (which is ultimately raised through taxation) expects that this will eventually lead to an increased level of profitability in the industry invested in or a reduction in another intervention that may be involved. The eradication of a disease in the farm animal population may lead to improved profitability and a more robust farming system. With zoonotic disease this may protect the human population and reduce treatment costs associated with protecting or treating people affected by these conditions. Enforcing microchipping may reduce the costs associated with lost dogs as they will allow a rapid tracing and return of the dog to owners. The same can be stated for microchipping horses where loose animals are a problem such as in Wales.

WHO SHOULD PAY?

Governments take in a lot of money from taxation of the general population and the demands on these resources are extensive, with everything from defence to education requiring government investment.

Cost-sharing is an attempt to ensure that those who need to will benefit, while ensuring that animal keepers are not unduly burdened by legislation that will help the public but would not be an automatic decision to carry out by the owner.

 Whether it is appropriate for government to invest is something that is debated with every initiative. Where there is a clear public health benefit then it is a relatively simple decision, as is the case with bovine tuberculosis. Where there is a disease of production such as bovine viral diarrhoea, where there is no public health risk but investment in eradicating this disease but investment may help maintain an efficient agricultural industry providing jobs and contributing to food security for the country, then investing seems like the obvious choice.

In the UK there is a move to get those who are most likely to benefit to pay, and this is mostly discussed when the agricultural industry is involved. This is very similar to the concept of 'polluter pays' that is enacted in environmental legislation. Where animal health and welfare issues are involved, then veterinary surgeons will be involved in deciding the appropriate cost-sharing principles.

SUMMARY OF ECONOMIC ISSUES

There is little that is for free in the world today and the treatment of animals is no different. In the UK many people feel that the cost associated with veterinary medicine and treatment is too high. Comparison with the same procedures in the human field would suggest that it represents good value. The costs to train a veterinary surgeon approximate to those to train a medical doctor, and who bears the bulk of the cost of this training will depend on the situation and country the prospective veterinary student finds themselves in.

The price of a veterinary consultation is composed of advice, medicine and possibly surgical intervention. In addition, there are a number of supporting roles in the veterinary practice that no practice could function without and these will be paid for by the fees generated by veterinary surgeons. Production of animal medicine will also require that the cost–benefit ratio is considered in order to maintain a profitable business. This can be at the group, farm and national levels. Some companion animal issues such as pet passports and quarantine legislation may require similar thinking.

Wherever the veterinary surgeon finds themselves working then the economics will be important. All of veterinary medicine requires resources and these have to be effectively managed, whether it is to produce a profitable practice or to manage the resources of a charity or government department in order to produce the best outcome for all those involved – owners, animals and many other stakeholders.

8
VETS AND ETHICS

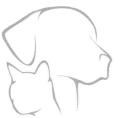

KEY POINTS

- There are many frameworks that Veterinary Surgeons can use to think about ethics.

- Always be honest and open – even when it may cause personal difficulty.

- There are many ethical issues and changing uses of animals will cause more.

- No one view is agreed by all veterinary surgeons.

The profession of being a veterinary surgeon is one that is intimately linked with ethics. This includes both their professional ethics and the personal ethics that they may bring to the profession. These can be from religious backgrounds or from detailed personal questioning of the issues that occur in daily life. Ethics in this context is wider than the welfare of animals that is dealt with elsewhere in this book. It is how we conduct ourselves as a profession, how society uses and interacts with animals and how the profession interacts with society.

VETS AND ETHICS

Ethical thinking is a way of thinking about the reasons behind why things are morally right or wrong. The study of ethics and an appreciation of the framework of ideas underpin the decision to decide that an action performed or not-performed on an animal is correct. Examples of such questions might be the decision to euthanase an animal, to conduct research using an animal, to campaign throughout society for a change or to become involved in a specific part of the career. For some, consideration of ethics may lead to a decision to leave the career due to personal changes or changes in the wider society. The decisions that are made depend on how the veterinary surgeon thinks, but there are many schools of ethics that allow a disciplined thought process to be applied. Two examples of ethical frameworks are the consequential theories where decisions are based on actions that produce the best outcome for all involved; this might be the case where society decides that a particular approach is taken, such as badger culling in the UK or invasive species control in wildlife conservation such as removing black rats from Anacapa Island in the USA. The second example of an ethical framework is deontological, where the ethical status (good or bad) is based on the actions of the person involved and their duties are assessed rather than the outcomes. Following the rules of a professional body is the desirable behaviour. So even if the outcome is less than desired, as long as the rules are followed then the behaviour is still assessed as morally correct. Other ethical frameworks are used as well.

Honesty and openness

One of the underlying principles of veterinary medicine is that the practitioners should be open and honest with their clients and society as a whole. This can be difficult as it means that mistakes by either the veterinary surgeon or a colleague should be confessed in order to preserve the reputation of the veterinary surgeon and the profession as a whole.

VETS AND THE USE OF ANIMALS

Humans have used animals throughout history and animals play a role in all societies. These roles are as food, as part of a herding or hunting team, as companions, as status symbols and as research tools, as well as other reasons that are less easily defined. As society has progressed and become more thoughtful about the use of animals, ethical considerations have become more discussed. The use of animals as food is probably the oldest use of animals, although companion animals may be of similar vintage.

To produce animals for food requires that some will have to be killed in order to provide food and other components such as leather. Milk and wool also require that animals are bred with specific characteristics, and males may later be surplus to requirements and removed from the herd as meat animals or low-value waste animals. There are two manners in which it is possible to look at this; it can be considered that vets by being involved in the food production industry are protecting the welfare and ensuring that the animals in the industry have the best life. By doing this it is also an efficient system so only the minimal number of animals is used to produce the food required. Another point of view is that by entering the industry, they are facilitating the system. By having vets involved with the perception of caring for animals it allows the industry to continue with its exploitation of animals. Vets can take either position and come to a decision about whether they decide to work in the sector. In a similar way, many people have issues with the equine racing industry, with an increasing awareness of horseracing deaths and injuries. In addition to this there are issues with the use of whips and the amount of animals that are bred and fail to become racing successes.

USING WHIPS ON HORSES?

Whips are used in racing to encourage the horse during a race and can be used to direct the animal away from danger. The use of a whip is associated with pain.

Is it right that we strike animals? The racing industry is placing them in a position that the horses may not choose if given a free choice. Should pain be used to make an animal race faster or should it be placed in a position where it is in danger? Can we use a whip sometimes but not others?

The veterinary surgeon involved in the equine racing industry faces a similar issue to the vet involved in food production. They can be regarded as protecting the welfare of the animals involved, but they can also be considered as facilitating the industry in allowing the animals to race to the animals' own detriment. Inappropriate treatment in the racing industry has been highlighted – including the misuse of drugs to mask pain or modify behaviour by increasing the horse's awareness, relaxing the animal or improving the airway efficiency of the animal.

As discussed before, when a vet is treating the animal, there is always a potential for adverse effects. This means that the use of a large range of substances is banned by the racing industry to protect the welfare of the animal; for example, after administration of a pain-controlling drug, horses may exacerbate a prior injury that leads to permanent damage. Alongside this there is the issue of fairness in the race, with trainers and owners attempting to gain an advantage. How involved the veterinary surgeon becomes depends on the perception of the ethical issues involved. In some very rare cases there may be veterinary surgeons that are totally complicit in supplying and administering banned drugs to horses and this will break professional rules and put the health of the animals at risk. However, there are issues for the vets that work in the industry to consider such as the fate of unsuccessful animals and the training regimes that they are under. There are unsurprisingly only a few animals that will make it to the racing track. Many will be eliminated for poor performance on the way through to the racing track. It is a thought for the professional veterinary surgeon involved in the industry to consider.

In the companion animal industry there are similar issues related to the use that society puts to the animals. Companion animals are bred to meet the expectations of owners such as looks, ability to work, prize-winning potential or preservation of traditional breeds. Status is also an important reason for people acquiring animals; these can be fighting dogs used to defend the owner or a breed or species that is associated with celebrity owners. Breeds have been developed from similar looking individuals to the current shapes that range from small Chihuahua dogs to large bulldogs. The shape of the breeds can lead to heads that are too large for the pelvic canal of the mothers and lead to an increased requirement for caesarean sections. Other breeds have difficulty breathing due to the anatomy of the head and neck and other breeds have mobility issues all due to breeding changes.

PEDIGREE DOGS

Breeding pedigree animals that win prizes gives satisfaction to many people and many enjoy watching the shows where they are exhibited. To win prizes means conforming to the standards – but what if the standards produce animals that are not healthy? Should veterinary surgeons be involved or should we place limits, such as neutering animals that are diagnosed with hereditary problems? Or should we not treat these animals at all if we do not agree with showing? Which would be the more consistently ethical approach?

Unusual species also are attractive to owners due to the status that is accrued to them due to their unique status. The requirements for care are frequently complex and poorly understood by either the owner or the wider community of vets and experts. This will lead to poor welfare of animals and birds kept in captivity as pets due to the lack of knowledge available.

For the vet there are a number of ethical issues and a number of levels at which the ethics may be considered. In all situations, the individual animal must be protected from further harm and the options of treatment, surgery and euthanasia. The owner may require advice and further education in order to maintain the welfare of the animal. Treatment of the animals in this case may perpetuate the issue within a species or breed. In all species a reliance on caesarean sections to allow breeding (Belgian blue cattle, Texel sheep, bulldogs) may lead to further interventions within the group of animals and perpetuating the requirement for caesarean sections. The question has to be asked in all these cases is whether the vet should take additional action (neutering, give the owner advice) to minimise this issue.

Exotic species (reptiles, birds, some mammal species) will require treatment in many cases. Treating these animals will protect their welfare as will adding to the owners' knowledge or developing the knowledge through research to keep these animals. However, as a professional body, the promotion of treatment of exotic species will give legitimacy to keeping these species and – as with all of the sectors that vets are involved in – will require consideration by the vet about their personal ethics and what they want to achieve and are comfortable about supporting.

If the use of animals is a continuous line with the use of these for food production at one end the other is that society should not be using animals at all. Organisations and people who hold this view suggest that any use of animals is akin to slavery and this includes the use of animals as pets. The suggestion is that the practice of pet-owning is inappropriate and should be phased out.

VETS AND WIDER SOCIETY

By keeping animals, society has to consider the ethical issues; some of these are individual matters but others are decided at a society level. Veterinary surgeons are at the forefront of discussing these matters and helping society as a whole to come to the decision about important animal matters. Matters that might be considered as a society include animal testing, the carrying out of routine mutilations, how animals are kept and for what purposes, and how we interact with wildlife throughout the world.

Research is an important undertaking and an area where many veterinary surgeons work developing new knowledge. In research there is sometimes a need to test new treatments, understand mechanisms of disease or normal functions, validate tests or prevention strategies. It is possible to partially answer these questions in systems that do not involve live animals but there is a wide-ranging debate about the point at which live animal use should be curtailed. An example of a vet involved in the public debate about the use of animals is Andrew Knight who wrote *The Costs and Benefits of Animal Experiments* and has campaigned on a number of animal welfare issues worldwide. He has a detailed website outlining his views on these and other issues (www.andrewknight.info). This vet has put considerable effort into developing his own ethical framework and is putting it into the public view in an attempt to influence the debate and produce change at a societal level. His position is that live animals are too frequently used in experimentation and other alternatives should be explored. This is expressed by the research community by the phrase 'reduce, refine and replace'. Animal experiments should be done as infrequently as possible, with as few animals as possible. Where possible, other techniques should be used to explore questions of interest to scientists. Vets who support animal research are more reluctant to speak out, as this position is associated with potential for threats. For an alternative point of view, Adrian Morrison wrote *An Odyssey with Animals* exploring the alternative point of view. There will be considerable debate about this for many years yet and the answer will change depending on how technology and society changes. These changes will be influenced by the voices of a large variety of people. Veterinary surgeons with their training in scientific investigation and welfare are particularly well placed to provide important insights for policymakers and assisting in developing legislation that is underpinned by good ethical and scientific thinking in this matter.

A treatment for Alzheimer's in people is being developed. To validate this test requires implants to be placed in the brains of rhesus macaques. The animals will be returned to consciousness so that when the treatment is administered the response in the brain can be monitored. Is this permissible in your view? How likely should success be and how many animals are acceptable and what effect would you expect in the people that finally get the drug?

There are a number of mutilations that are carried out on animals. These are changes to the anatomy of the animal carried out for reasons of safety, convenience or aesthetics as required by the owner. As with all of these issues, the vet can refuse or agree to carry out these changes on the individual animal depending on the vets.

Such issues might be castration of males, removal of horns in cattle or beaks from poultry. Tails can be removed in sheep, dogs and pigs. The cropping of ears of pedigree dogs is carried out in some countries including the United States, as is declawing. Devocalisation is carried out on dogs in many states in the United States quite legally, although some states have made it illegal. There are many more of these interventions carried out throughout the world and many of them are only possible with veterinary intervention.

Discussion regarding the necessity for some of these procedures and whether there should be legislation to prohibit them is a discussion that should be held in public. In the UK, the farm animal welfare committee frequently coordinates this discussion. This group is chaired by a highly experienced veterinary surgeon and past president of the Royal College of Veterinary Surgeons (RCVS). With the group of veterinary surgeons, farmers and scientists, the discussion of farm animal welfare is kept under review. The companion animal discussion in the UK is guided by the Companion Animal Welfare Council, chaired by Lord Soulsby, carries out the function of discussing the relevance of legislation and welfare standards for companion animals. The Welsh Animal Health and Welfare Framework has responsibility for both companion and farm as well as wild animals. This group gains veterinary advice from a well-respected practitioner and the chief veterinary officer. In all these cases the vets will work with other interested people to thrash out the ethical issues and complexities of managing farm animals.

It is not only through the government channels that vets attempt to influence the discussion of the ethics around keeping animals. A veterinary surgeon is director of campaigns at Compassion in World Farming to promote that organisation's vision of good farming.

So vets are interacting with many members of society (sometimes referred to as stakeholders), balancing the needs of the animal at the time it is seen with its needs later in life. The immediate treatment of the animal may not be to its benefit but the long-term risks incurred by not doing the intervention may make the intervention worthwhile. Alternatively the intervention may well be to the animal's benefit at the time but may lead to a poorer outcome on the long term for the animal or for the breed (or species). The use of caesarean sections to allow the animals to give birth will allow the mother and offspring to thrive. However, it may lead to further breeding episodes and further surgery to allow breeding.

There are also considerations about the interaction with wildlife. This can be human–wildlife interaction such as elephants raiding crops. Ethical considerations may involve culling of individual animals in order to keep the local population from killing a lot more animals and endangering the species as a whole. Capture and removal may be an alternative but it may reduce the resources for other initiatives. All of these issues will have to be balanced within a defensible ethical framework. Badger–cattle interactions are a similar UK issue, and the issues have been replicated across the world as vets are involved in the attempt to control tuberculosis in the cattle population. Bovine TB causes disease in many species including humans, and the control measures in place are to minimise and eliminate the disease burden on the human population. In Australia, wild buffalo also carried the disease along with feral (escaped) cattle and in New Zealand the common brushtail possum carries the disease and transmits it to cattle. While the wildlife (badgers, possums, buffalo) are not owned in a conventional sense, they do need to be considered in the control of a disease that affects all the wider range of species. This has caused considerable debate in the UK. The badger is an iconic wild mammal in the UK countryside and its control has proved controversial. The vets at the British Veterinary Association, the British Cattle Veterinary Association and the Veterinary Association for Wildlife Management have made significant representations to government in an attempt to balance the needs of farmers to continue working, minimise the disease in cattle and the culling required and protect the welfare of the badgers. There is again active debate about the approach, with opposing groups looking towards cattle controls and vaccination of badgers and cattle being advocated. Ethical issues that are considered when discussing control of bovine TB include the impact on the business of the farmers that provides for their livelihood. The disease, if uncontrolled, will have welfare impacts as cattle suffer the disease and the current controls require culling (killing) of animals that are tested as having the disease. Badgers (and other infected wildlife) will probably have clinical signs associated with the disease. The current options require culling of the wildlife involved in transmitting the disease and novel interventions will impose a cost on the individual animals. The evidence of harm and benefit for each of these elements needs to be carefully assessed. It is not going to be a decision completely made by veterinary surgeons but they will be critical in advancing the debate.

Wild animals are also kept in zoos and in circuses. The ethical debate around keeping animals in both of these systems is also a matter of intense public debate. The cost and benefits are evaluated in a similar manner to the debates about other issues. Zoos provide a place where people can see these animals that might be impossible otherwise. The animals will be protected from predators and starvation but these basic protections may be the only advantages with natural behaviours such as the predatory behaviour of big cats being impossible to allow. These compromises are imposed on animals by keeping them in zoos, and veterinary surgeons that work in these facilities must be comfortable with that.

In all cases, as part of a veterinary surgeon's training, the ability to bring a structured thought process and fit the relevant facts and opinions into a framework to bring about the best solutions is essential.

VETS AND RELIGION

Religious issues impact on the treatment of animals. These can be issues from the country where the vet is practising or the vet's own attitudes. The legislation in the country may clash with the religious and cultural values of part of the population. In some cases, veterinary surgeons may receive guidance and support from the edicts of their religions.

Religions generally give guidance on how people should behave and some of these rules discuss how animals are seen in the context of the worldview and should be treated. In the Christian Bible, the Genesis story speaks about 'dominion over the fish of the sea, and over the fowl of the air, and over the cattle, and over all the earth, and over every creeping thing that creepeth upon the earth'. Buddhism, Hinduism and Jainism regard animals as having souls that at least have the potential to become human. Almost all faiths advocate kindness to animals as part of the text, although culture and interpretation may change the delivery. Judaism and Islam both advocate for the kind treatment of animals and in Judaism vegetarianism is the first dietary law, although slaughter of animals is allowed under strict rules and this has similarities to Islamic halal slaughter rules.

Vets with a strong Christian faith would advocate that their faith guides them and that it will reinforce the strong integrity that they already have as a veterinary surgeon. This attitude is echoed by vets from all faiths who frequently cite guidance from their faith as a strong influence on their work.

Religious laws in some areas in the world may cause welfare issues that conflict with the beliefs of the practicing veterinarian. Hinduism does advocate kindness to animals and cattle in particular will be cared for. Euthanasia is, however, difficult due to Hinduism requiring that cattle are not killed. This will sometime lead an animal to suffer for a prolonged period of time when euthanasia would be in the animals' welfare. For a vet (and particularly a Western-trained veterinary surgeon), this can be very frustrating.

The most controversial issue when religion and animals are discussed is the slaughter of animals as food. Both Islam and Judaism have specific rules for the slaughter of animals. It is likely that these rules were put in place historically as the best way of ensuring that food was safe for people to eat. However, these would be superseded in the opinion of many. In 2014, the president elect of the British Veterinary Association was the public face of a new wave of publicity to have non-stun slaughter banned in the UK. For many there is real difficulty in this as it is seen as an attack on the faith of a minority population. As with many of the issues, a rigorous ethical framework is key to maintaining a rational debate. Issues in religious slaughter are the suffering of animals as they are bled to death while conscious. This has to be balanced against the requirement of society to allow the free practice of religion. In halal slaughter (for Islamic customers), stunning may be permitted and for most this is sufficient to solve the problem. Shechita slaughter (for Jewish customers) does not permit stunning and proponents suggest that the loss of consciousness is faster than other accepted methods. Whether it is permissible to interfere with the practice of a religion is – as with other issues discussed here – not a decision that will be made by vets alone but veterinary surgeons will be key to the discussions around religious slaughter.

ETHICS IN VETERINARY MEDICINE

The rules of behaviour applied to veterinary medicine are referred to as 'veterinary ethics'. Ethics is a branch of philosophy that is concerned with correct behaviour. The study and application of ethics helps ensure that the rules developed by individuals, the professional bodies and society as a whole are developed from a rigorous framework.

The discussions about ethics will vary in the detail but all will be around the benefits to the animal and the detrimental effects and in a similar vein the detriment and benefits to wider groups species and society as a whole.

All vets will have a personal underlying philosophy and many of these will be related to their religion. Some can find this enormously useful and use it to help their practice. Like all things, however, it is not always helpful and welfare issues around slaughter will remain contentious.

Whatever the ethical issues under discussion, with their expertise in welfare and medicine, vets should remain at the heart of the matter.

9

VETERINARY SURGEONS AND WELFARE

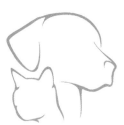

> ## KEY POINTS
>
> - Veterinary surgeons swear an oath to protect animal welfare.
> - The definition of good welfare is difficult to determine but good welfare is easy to recognize.
> - Good welfare is indicative of a good society.
> - Euthanasia is a good welfare outcome in some cases.
> - Measuring and preventing welfare compromises is becoming more important.

INTERNATIONAL VETERINARY OATHS

Almost all veterinary surgeons will cite animal welfare as their main motivation and members of the public will expect animal welfare to be placed above all else. Almost all professional organisations have welfare as a priority for their members. In order to emphasise this to the members and the public, organisations will ask those joining to swear an oath that states their underlying philosophy. Welfare is stated as a guiding principle in many veterinary oaths and some of the oaths are written below.

Australia

I solemnly swear to practice veterinary science ethically and conscientiously for the benefit of animal welfare, animal and human health, users of veterinary services and the community. I will endeavour to maintain my practice of veterinary science to current professional standards and will strive to improve my skills and knowledge through continuing professional development. I acknowledge that along with the privilege of acceptance into the veterinary profession comes community and professional responsibility. I will maintain these principles throughout my professional life.

Canada

As a member of the veterinary medical profession, I solemnly swear that I will use my scientific knowledge and skills for the benefit of society. I will strive to promote animal health and welfare, relieve animal suffering, protect the health of the public and environment, and advance comparative medical knowledge. I will practise my profession conscientiously, with dignity, and in keeping with the principles of veterinary medical ethics. I will strive continuously to improve my professional knowledge and competence and to maintain the highest professional and ethical standards for myself and the profession.

India

Being admitted to the profession of veterinary medicine, I solemnly swear to use my scientific knowledge and skill for the benefit of society through the protection of animal health and welfare, the prevention and relief of animal suffering, the conservation of livestock resources, the promotion of public health and the advancement of medical knowledge. I will practice my profession conscientiously, with dignity and in keeping with the principles of veterinary medical ethics. I accept as a lifelong obligation the continual improvement of my professional knowledge and competence.

Ireland

I solemnly and sincerely declare that I will, to the best of my ability, uphold the honour, dignity and integrity of the veterinary profession, that I will promote the welfare of animals entrusted to my care and that I will abide by the rulings of the Veterinary Council.

Philippines

Being admitted to the profession of veterinary medicine, I solemnly swear to use my scientific knowledge and skills for the benefit of society through the protection of animal health, the relief of animal suffering, the conservation of animal resources, the promotion of public health, and the advancement of medical knowledge. I will practice my profession conscientiously, with dignity, and in keeping with the principles of veterinary medical ethics. I accept as a lifelong obligation the continual improvement of my professional knowledge and competence.

Sri Lanka

Being admitted to the profession of veterinary medicine, I solemnly swear to use my scientific knowledge and skills for the benefit of society through the protection of animal health, the relief of animal suffering, the conservation of livestock resources, the promotion of public health and the advancement of medical knowledge. I will practice my profession conscientiously, with dignity and in keeping with the principles of veterinary medical ethics. I accept as a lifelong obligation the continual improvement of my professional knowledge and competence.

Taiwan

Having chosen veterinary medicine to be my profession, I hereby solemnly swear that I will treat my teachers with reverence and my colleagues with comity; that I will devote my professional knowledge and skills to the respect of animal life, the protection of animal health, the relief of animal suffering, the conservation of livestock resources, the promotion of public health and the advancement of medical knowledge; and that I will collaborate with human medical professionals for the benefit of society. I will strive to improve relations between man and animals, societal harmony, and the protection of our environment, and to maintain the highest professional and ethical standards for the profession. I will practice my profession with good conscience, dignity, morality, and professional ethics. I will endeavour continuously to advance my professional knowledge and competence. Upon my beliefs stated above, I hereby solemnly and voluntarily pledge my oath.

UK

I promise and solemnly declare that I will pursue the work of my profession with integrity and accept my responsibilities to the public, my clients, the profession and the Royal College of Veterinary Surgeons and that above all my constant endeavour will be to ensure the health and welfare of animals committed to my care.

USA

Being admitted to the profession of veterinary medicine, I solemnly swear to use my scientific knowledge and skills for the benefit of society through the protection of animal health and welfare, the prevention and relief of animal suffering, the conservation of animal resources, the promotion of public health, and the advancement of medical knowledge. I will practice my profession conscientiously, with dignity, and in keeping with the principles of veterinary medical ethics. I accept as a lifelong obligation the continual improvement of my professional knowledge and competence.

WHAT IS WELFARE?

Animal welfare is the assessment of the wellbeing of animals. At its core is the fact that animals are sentient beings in their own right with the ability to feel and therefore have the right not to have unnecessary pain and suffering inflicted upon them. Much discussion has been centred on defining pain and suffering in animals.

Do animals feel pain?

The question of whether animals feel pain has been debated for hundreds of years with intense debate about the treatment of animals being found in the treatises of Pythagoras and Aristotle. The views presented by these two important philosophers took opposing views on the utility of animals. Pythagoras believed that animals had a soul similar to humans and should be treated in some ways as equals. Aristotle believed that animals were lower than humans and therefore did not need to be treated with as much consideration as humans. A student of Aristotle, Theophrastus argued that animals feel and suffer as humans but due to the unearthing and dissemination of Aristotle's writing by Thomas Aquinas in the eleventh century this view of animals as things to use was widely accepted for many centuries. Descartes expanded on this view and argued that animals were essentially robots with all explanations for animal behaviour being mechanistic in nature. With support from this philosophy by such an influential philosopher building on the ideas of an older and arguably even more influential philosopher, these ideas were generally accepted by Western society and scientists until relatively recently. A modern philosopher that has challenged that view is Peter Singer, who suggests that as we can see responses analogous to those that we would associate with pain in ourselves, we cannot justifiably state that animals cannot feel pain.

WHAT IS PAIN?

All people have experienced pain but what is it exactly? That is a more complex question than might first be thought as it has both a physical and an emotional component with acute and chronic attributes. It can be protective or damaging dependent on the situation. The pain of, for example, a cut in the skin results from the activation of pain receptors in the tissues and these can respond to thermal, mechanical and chemical insults. These nerves are termed 'nociceptors' and receptors at the terminal end of the nerves respond to one or more of these stimuli resulting in an electrical signal along the axon termed an 'action potential'. Transmission of the action potential through chemical signalling using neurotransmitters to other nerves will allow the brain to sense the insult. With reflex actions there will then be a rapid response such as withdrawal of the limb that suffers a burn.

If we assume that animals are not automatons then there will be a psychological component to pain. The animal suffering this insult will learn to avoid situations that result in a painful outcome. This will be useful in avoiding further injury in the animal's life.

Physiological signals that may indicate a painful issue include an increase in heart rate, breathing rate, blood pressure, vocalization and behavioural changes associated with that species.

Long term – chronic – pain can, be a problem for the animal as it may change the animal's response to its environment. Chronic pain may well reduce the awareness of the animal, change its attitude (the animal may become more reclusive or it may become more aggressive), reduce its desire to eat and drink or interact with other animals in its group. This may be associated with a reduction in production but it is sometimes astounding the conditions that animals will reproduce and grow in. Cattle can be farmed with severe lameness and still become pregnant and milk. It is part of the veterinary surgeon's task to determine where the pain is occurring and alleviate it, along with educating owners who may not realise the animal is in pain and what reductions in the animal's performance the pain is causing, whether it is in the many cases of farm animals or with the pet dog that is suffering from advanced arthritis.

Being pain-free is not the only criterion that is considered for good welfare. The definition of good welfare is hotly debated and there have been many attempts to find a comprehensive definition. Attempts include suggesting that the animal should have a good life, or how the animal is coping with the environment it finds itself in. Each definition has its detractors and supporters and each will have an application to a specific situation. Whatever the specific definition, there has to be a framework that guides veterinary surgeons (and others) in deciding whether an animal's welfare needs are being met.

THE FIVE FREEDOMS

A commonly accepted framework for veterinary Surgeons to work under is the Five Freedoms. Derived from a concept first suggested by Professor Brambell in 1965 and further developed by the Farm Animal Welfare Council, the Five Freedoms are:

- Freedom from hunger or thirst by ready access to fresh water and a diet to maintain full health and vigour.

- Freedom from discomfort by providing an appropriate environment including shelter and a comfortable resting area.

- Freedom from pain, injury or disease by prevention or rapid diagnosis and treatment.

- Freedom to express (most) normal behaviour by providing sufficient space, proper facilities and company of the animal's own kind.

- Freedom from fear and distress by ensuring conditions and treatment that avoid mental suffering.

How are they measured?

The Five Freedoms give the veterinary surgeon a toolbox of thoughts to judge the welfare of animals that have been placed under their care. In order to apply these, the veterinary surgeon has to assess specific factors in order to determine specific problems and to give advice to correct them as well as to provide evidence that may result in prosecution.

Freedom from hunger and thirst may be obvious in extreme cases as starvation due to food withholding by the owner but looking at the body condition score of animals may reveal a more insidious lack of food. However, the freedom refers to a diet that maintains full health and vigour and overfeeding is as much a welfare problem as underfeeding. Dogs are predominantly the species that are overfed and this can cause other health issues with arthritis and heart and breathing problems being the most likely. Although obesity is simply the supply of more calories than required by the animal, the reasons for this oversupply of calories in companion animals are probably as complex as the reasons in the human field. Emotional bonds may influence the feeding habits; the owners may genuinely not see the animal as fat and there may be psychological or physical illness on the owner's part that contributes to the overfeeding. There are cases where elderly people with age-related mental issues will overfeed animals and cause obesity: this is a welfare issue as animals in these homes are loved by the owners but will suffer from pressure-associated ulcers, arthritis and other issues. It can be difficult for the veterinary surgeon involved. Carers such as children and grandchildren may have to be involved to help manage the situation and other (human) health providers may have an influence on the case management.

An appropriate diet is also dependent on the appropriate composition, and what this is for companion animals – in particular dogs – is debated the world over. Raw diets are advocated by many veterinary surgeons, trainers and owners as the preferred option due to the health advantages, particularly dental health advantages. In other species (such as exotic animals), the provision of a suitable diet may be difficult, require complex preparations and may not be completely understood.

The environment in which an animal is kept will influence its mental health and wellbeing. The basic maintenance of an animal's accommodation should prevent injury. The bedding provided should be safe and encourage resting. The freedom from discomfort has a lot of overlap with the freedom to express normal behaviour.

Probably the most high-profile situation where the environment of the animal is concerned are battery cages. Battery cages restrict the movement of the inhabitants and allow the birds to be kept in higher numbers in an equivalent space to other systems (higher stocking density) and for a lower cost. Opponents argue that the hens kept in these situations are not able to flap and move around and so exhibit signs of boredom such as picking at their feathers.

Although battery hen systems have been banned in the European Union, it still remains a common egg production system in the rest of the world – but the proportion is slowly reducing. Hens are not the only animals kept in battery cages. Chinese farms keep sun bears for bile, while mink are kept in similar cages, as are civets for coffee production in Southeast Asia and foxes for fur farming.

The environmental compromises that may be made to keep animals are sometimes less obvious. Zoo and aquarium creatures are kept in conditions that many find unacceptable. Some animals in their natural environment would travel many kilometres. The opinion of many people – including some veterinary surgeons – is that it is impossible to keep, for example, killer whales, dolphins, cheetahs and elephants in conditions that allow them to be comfortable, express normal behaviour and live an acceptable life. In companion animals, the exotic species may suffer from similar conditions; for example, parrot owners may not be able to provide sufficient ranges with enough enrichment to allow the birds to demonstrate the inquisitive and exploratory behaviour that characterises these highly intelligent animals.

Where a veterinary surgeon may well be thought to be central to the Five Freedoms is to provide accurate, rapid and appropriate treatment. However, the animal does need to be presented to the veterinary surgeon to allow this to happen. In the UK, the animal welfare legislation has been altered to support this and make it an owner's responsibility to seek help for the animals under their care. The owner obviously needs to spot and acknowledge that the animal needs veterinary care. It is possible that many owners will get used to slow onset conditions and not realise there is a problem. This can be in both individual and group situations.

The freedom from fear and distress requires a good understanding of the fear responses of the species. This fear may be caused by the presence of predators or by unusual noises. Slaughterhouses are probably where this is most considered and many are designed to minimise the fear and distress to the animals going through the facility. Poor treatment in many forms can cause fear and distress, such as frequent physical chastisement to companion animals and this would be a welfare issue; detecting it may take skill on the part of the veterinary surgeon or welfare inspector, especially where it is being deliberately hidden.

ANIMAL WELFARE – NOT JUST ABOUT ANIMALS

Animal welfare and cruelty to animals is not just about the animal. The way society treats animals is seen as an indicator on how civilised a society is by some commentators and many animal rights organisations.

In other cases, animal cruelty will indicate problems with people more directly. The link between animal cruelty and child and domestic abuse is increasingly being recognised, while cruelty to animals by children can be evidence of abuse of the children or of other abuse in the home. Animals that are abused are more likely to bite the owners or children. In some cases it may be an early indicator of abuse in a household. This link is recognised in both the USA with the National Research Center on the Link between Violence to People and Animals and in the UK by the Domestic Abuse Veterinary Initiative.

Key to dealing with this issue is recognising the signs of animal abuse in a domestic environment. It is important that the veterinary surgeon considers and recognises non-accidental injuries; these are injuries that, when considered carefully, do not fit the history. These are difficult for veterinary surgeons to recognise, as many cannot conceive of deliberate harm, but once these have been identified it is probably a social good that action is taken. The veterinary surgeon is not expected to solve the problem, but consideration should be given to reporting the issue. As an ethical issue, this has to be balanced against client confidentiality.

ASSURANCE SCHEMES

The welfare of production animals is a concern for large sections of the public, with welfare being reported as a major purchasing decision when choosing food. To address this there are assurance schemes that check welfare standards. UK consumers are familiar with the Red Tractor scheme and Freedom Foods, while in the USA there are many organisations that fill the same niche including Food Alliance, Animal Welfare Approved, Certified Humane and others.

These schemes look at a number of things in order to assure the public that food purchased is from animals that have been kept in a manner that the public would find acceptable. Assurance schemes will look at the space allowances for the animals and the standard of maintenance in the accommodation. The farm will also be assessed for how many animals die (mortality rate) and how many are sick (morbidity rate); other factors that are considered important are the health of young animals, lameness in the animals and mastitis. These criteria have been developed in partnership with veterinary surgeons but often the input of a veterinary surgeon is required to develop the detailed health plans that are part of assurance plans. This involves taking the data from the farmers' records and the veterinary surgeon's knowledge of the farm. They may be working to modify the flow of cattle to the milking parlour to minimise lameness in the dairy herds, or producing vaccination plans preventing pneumonia in beef calves.

Farm assurance schemes in the past would concentrate on documentary evidence, including fairly static measurements such as the amount of space available for an animal to lie in. This was of benefit as it helped to drive improvements but is sometimes considered peripheral to the effect on animals. As the farm assurance schemes have developed, outcome-based measures are more important. This will involve the collation of welfare-associated data on the farm. This could be mastitis (udder infection) numbers in the herd, lameness in the flock or tail-biting in pigs. The veterinary surgeon will be sitting with the farmer and looking at areas of concern that can be drawn out from this data collection.

The quality of the advice given will be heavily reliant on the data that this advice is based on; this is a major potential drawback for the assurance schemes. Independent audit does address this to some degree and those assurance schemes that are moving to outcome-based systems incorporate independent checking. Veterinary surgeons involved in these schemes will be encouraging the farmer in collecting the relevant and accurate data. The accurate identification of key issues will benefit the farmer and his animals and at the moment there are no prescriptive targets for any welfare measurement. These may be instituted to further drive welfare improvements but this will probably prove controversial if it is instituted.

Farm assurance schemes, with all their limitations, are at least schemes that monitor welfare and drive improvements. The equine and companion animal areas have no equivalent organisations. It may not be appropriate to assess cat and dog owners in the same way but the welfare of these animals is obviously as important.

HOW IS THE WELFARE OF ANIMALS PROTECTED?

The welfare of all animals is protected in law all across the world. Enforcing these laws falls to a variety of bodies with powers to prosecute those that cause cruelty in animals. The Animal and Plant Health Agency (APHA , formerly the Animal Health and Veterinary Laboratory Agency) will monitor the welfare of animals through its staff and bring about prosecutions. Charitable organisations such as the RSPCA in England and Wales will bring about prosecutions. The SSPCA will prosecute in Scotland. In the USA, the USDA will carry out inspections and give advice regarding animal welfare violations; if these pieces of advice are not taken on board then prosecution may result. Other charitable organisations in the USA will also carry out prosecutions on behalf of animals.

In most countries there are both governmental organisations and charitable organisations that will bring about prosecutions within their borders. These organisations will use veterinary expertise in order to develop the policies, gather evidence of the clinical issues and produce educational materials that may help owners to avoid inadvertent welfare problems.

WHAT WELFARE ISSUES REMAIN?

Animal welfare has improved since the first animal charities with an interest in preventing cruelty were set up and interest in the welfare of animals has increased since Ruth Harrison published *Animal Machines* in 1964. Animal welfare has slowly been improved as scientific knowledge has increased and education has disseminated this knowledge to a wider audience. Successes have been long and hard fought for and need to be maintained. The slow withdrawal of battery cages in egg production is a good example of progress in improving the welfare of farmed livestock. Changes to the care of animals before and during research procedures is another improvement in welfare that has occurred since society's general interest in the welfare of animals has increased. What welfare concerns catch the public's interest is going to vary on many factors. These will include the media's interest in the issues, whether other events interfere, the legislative bodies' desire to pursue a legal avenue, the scientific evidence available around the issues and competing viewpoints about the welfare of animals.

There are remaining issues that are believed by some to compromise the welfare of many species. Many of these issues are around mutilations permitted on animals both companion and farmed. Dogs, sheep and pigs all have had their tails docked by some owners. The justification for these amputations is the improvement in welfare due to a reduced chance of injury in the animals' future and to preserve the characteristics of the breed. Tail docking in dogs is carried out (where legal) in pups at one to four days old by placing an elastic band like those used in human dental braces around the tail. This blocks the blood flow to the tail and the unwanted tissue dies off.

The legal status of tail docking ranges from a total ban in Australia, restricted in England and Wales (Scotland legislated for a total ban) to countries where no legislation exists. The USA and Canada allows each state to decide on its own position. Opponents of tail docking in dogs argue that the removal of the tail is painful and of no benefit to the dog. The tail is an important communication mechanism in dogs and the removal of the tail carries the risk that the interaction with other dogs will be compromised. That balance in dogs may also be compromised by tail docking has been suggested. People who support tail docking would suggest that the removal of the tail is not painful in such young animals and could mean a more severe injury later in life is avoided. The hygiene of the dog is also suggested as a reason for the removal of tails. Tail length is also a characteristic of certain breeds such as German pointers or miniature schnauzers.

Whether tail docking will remain legal will depend on the influence of, among others, veterinary surgeons. Veterinary organisations have released statements about this matter. The BVA statement reads:

> The BVA is opposed to the docking of puppies' tails. BVA believes that puppies suffer unnecessary pain as a result of docking, and are deprived of a vital form of canine expression. Chronic pain can arise from poorly-performed docking.

> BVA would reiterate that surgical operations should not be undertaken unless necessary for therapeutic purposes and that docking should be banned as a procedure, other than for veterinary medical reasons, for all breeds of dog.

The AVMA opposes tail docking for cosmetic reasons and encourages the breed societies to remove the requirement for tail docking from the standards. Although the practice is banned totally in Australia, the AVA stance is similar. Both organisations also suggest that there is no positive reason to carry out the procedure. As a scientific profession, the veterinary organisations have also developed these positions based on the evidence base. There is no direct evidence of pain in new-born puppies but significant evidence of pain in new-born animals in other species is available. In the late nineteenth century it was believed that new-born children could not feel pain. It would appear the assumption that puppies will not feel pain is not as straightforward as it may appear to be. The level of injury to adult dogs with long tails is also unknown, with only a few limited studies about this. Where there is no specific legislation, the veterinary surgeons will have to make their own decisions about whether they can justify tail docking.

Dogs are not the only species that have their tail docked. Cattle, horses, sheep and pigs have all been routinely docked and still are in many places. The rationale for these procedures is to avoid injury and increase the hygiene of the animal. Lambs are docked to prevent fly strike in later life. Fly strike is a result of faecal soiling of the rear end of a sheep; this soiling frequently results from a parasite burden that is too high for the animal to cope with. Removal of the tail is carried out to prevent this, but pain at the time of docking has been well documented. Pigs will have their tails docked in the first week of life in order to reduce tail-biting in later life. Opponents of this would suggest that the tail-biting is due to poor husbandry in later life and the better option is to manage the animals appropriately as they grow.

Surgical interventions of all types are becoming less acceptable to society and slowly, as a result, the welfare regulations and codes are changing to reflect society. Different countries and areas are at different places in changing welfare. Surgical interventions apart from tail docking that are carried out are castration, ear cropping and debarking. These are all sometimes called surgical mutilations. Some of these interventions may have an overall beneficial effect while others are purely cosmetic in nature. Castration falls in the potentially beneficial category. Removal of the testicles will reduce inappropriate breeding and fighting between males. This is legally allowed in all countries but many organisations are reconsidering the necessity of castration. That it is a painful procedure is accepted but is the pain controllable and the overall benefit to the individual animal great enough to justify the intervention? That is a matter for the veterinary surgeon to discuss with the owner.

Cropping of ears is banned in many countries but it is still practised in the USA. This practice is the surgical remodelling of visible earflaps to produce a shape desired by the owner. This usually produces a pricked ear appearance. Veterinary ear cropping done under surgical conditions is unlikely to be severely painful but the intervention is unlikely to be of benefit. However, ear cropping is occasionally carried out by owners and in these cases the procedure may well be painful and cruel. The discussions about whether this will be allowed to continue will be influenced by discussions in society and once again veterinary organisations are influential in this debate. The AVMA opposes this, as do most other veterinary organisations throughout the world, as no benefit can be proven for the animal.

In the equine world, veterinary surgeons may well be asked to carry out firing of horse limbs or be asked to refer the animal to another practitioner. Firing of horses is the application of a red hot bar running around the leg or a pointed iron being punched into the tendon. The belief is that this will change the inflammation that has occurred as a result of an injury. This procedure is illegal in Australia and New Zealand but legal in most other countries – although the UK situation is a little more complex, with the RCVS suggesting that it is an unacceptable procedure. Veterinary surgeons will have to decide their position on whether to fire or to refer.

Not all of the welfare issues that remain (and there are many) are a result of direct interventions by owners, keepers or veterinary surgeons. The welfare of farm animals is a constant concern and a specific problem in both cattle and sheep. Cattle in the dairy industry are noted to be particularly lame as a group. Estimates vary but it is thought that about a quarter of cattle on some farms are lame. Veterinary surgeons are heavily involved in working to reduce lameness in the herd. This has been done in many ways. Veterinary surgeons worked with the industry to develop a way to measure the lameness that allowed simple comparisons between farms. The majority of lameness assessment is now done using the DairyCo mobility scoring system. A change in the attitude was also worked on by changing terminology from 'lameness', which has negative connotations, to 'mobility', which has more positive connotations. Mobility scoring has become more accepted as a management tool with the farming community, with cattle scored on a four-point scale. A cow scoring zero will move freely and walk with an even gait. Cattle scoring a one will have a slight restriction in the freedom of movement but no definite lameness. Score two cattle have a definite lameness on at least one leg and score three cattle are lame on at least one leg and unable to walk at the same speed as the rest of the herd. This system is easy to use and through this veterinary surgeons have worked with farmers to drive lameness down but there remains much work to be done. Most dairy cows will end their lives at an abattoir. Cattle being presented at an abattoir should not be lame and inspection of the animals is a responsibility of the veterinary surgeon at the abattoir. Should the animal be lame then a decision will be made whether to prosecute the owner or to give advice. This provides a further monitoring opportunity on the foot health of herds.

While the cattle industry does have an issue with lameness in the herd, a combination of initiatives are providing hope that this issue will be reduced in the future. By working with industry to develop a useable benchmarking initiative, this allows farmers to compare themselves to others and decide where they can improve. It can also assist by identifying lame cows rapidly so they can be treated quickly and are more likely to improve. Education of farmers regarding the impact of lame cows has helped to engage farmers with the issue. Farm assurance schemes have taken this issue on board and are asking farmers involved to record the level of mobility of their herd and this awareness combined with the education delivered through many avenues will hopefully improve the foot health of the farm.

If none of these work, prosecution under the relevant welfare legislation can be used. Lameness in the cattle herd is still too high in dairy cattle wherever they are kept but work from all these angles will – with time and good fortune – drive the amount down.

Lameness in the sheep flock is also an issue and has been identified by many organisations as such. The underlying causes of lameness in sheep may be different and the management options reflect this. The approaches to improving it are similar with identification of the problem, quantification of the problem, education of the farming and veterinary community. Prosecution is also used but generally as a last resort as where there are severe welfare problems it is common to find an underlying emotional, financial or mental health problem. Addressing these may produce a more satisfactory resolution for all concerned.

In all domestic species, humans have manipulated the genetics of animals on farms or as companions. This has been through choice of the males and females that are allowed to breed and has been sped up by artificial breeding techniques such as insemination and embryo transfer. This will produce characteristics that the people breeding these animals wish to see; these may be better food conversion in cattle, a change in the hip angle of dogs or changes in coat colour and pattern. There are many characteristics that have been bred into animals but while the breeder may desire them they may not be in the animal's best interests. Short-nosed breeds of animal may have difficulty breathing, hip angle may increase the chances of the animal becoming painfully lame and large birth weight or head size may lead to an increased chance of the need for caesarean section. Both farm and companion animals have issues associated with breeding choices. The veterinary organisations in many countries are working with breed societies to change the breed standards where the problem comes from the shape desired. German shepherds have been at the centre of work by veterinary surgeons and the Kennel Club of the UK to change the breeding policy from sloping backs (topline) to a more horizontal line to the back following public outcry when the BBC in *Pedigree Dogs Exposed* examined pedigree dog breeding. With other breeds, the ability to breathe has been compromised by a long-term shortening of the muzzle in brachycephalic (short-faced breeds) such as pugs and bulldogs.

Cat breeds such as the Scottish fold and Persian also have been bred with characteristics that are attractive to the breeders and buyers; the Scottish fold have a gene that promotes folding of the ear forwards, the Persian has breathing problems in the same manner as the brachycephalic dogs and the Scottish fold has a tendency to osteochondrodysplasia as a result of the breed character. These health issues have led to the breeds not being recognised for showing by many of the organizing bodies but not all of the cat societies have come to the same conclusion.

Some problems that have a genetic basis are more complex with multiple genes being involved. Working with veterinary surgeons, the breed societies are working to educate breeders and provide testing services as buyers of these animals ask for the animals to be tested in order to avoid the possible diseases.

Despite these initiatives there remains much work to be done in the pedigree dog world to reduce the welfare issues that are a result of breeding. Breeding for specific characteristics is not the only breeding problem. Irresponsible breeding can be uncontrolled breeding. Without homes for the young animals – whether they are kittens, puppies or foals – there will be welfare problems as abandonment increases alongside the need to euthanase more animals. Across most of the world, feral populations of dogs and cats are a problem. The welfare of these animals may be poor due to lack of care. In Wales, horses are frequently abandoned in fields – many as a result of overbreeding.

EUTHANASIA TO PROTECT THE WELFARE OF ANIMALS

The discussion so far has centred around the education or prosecution of the owner to prevent further welfare problems. The welfare of the animal directly involved must also be protected. In some cases the animal may be treatable and removing it from the situation and re-treating the animal may well be possible. These cases can be very satisfying to be involved in.

But in some cases treatment will be impossible, such as cattle with broken legs or dogs with severe untreated demodicosis (a difficult to treat mite disease). Where this is the case, then euthanasia may be a positive welfare outcome. Apart from ending the pain and suffering that the animal is feeling, euthanasing a suffering animal that the veterinary surgeon cannot effectively treat may allow more time and resources to be committed to other animals and increase the success rate for the treatment centre or situation.

THE FUTURE OF WELFARE

Changes in how we will keep animals as a society will occur over time and the impact on animal welfare is unknown. The meat consumption of the world is likely to increase, as is the desire to eat dairy products and drink milk. This will impact on wildlife as land is converted to food production. As medical knowledge advances then the ability to treat will increase and this will change our ability to affect the welfare of animals. Research will almost inevitably lead to experiments on animals being carried out. New exotic pets will become popular and require good management specific to their species and treatment. Other changes that cannot be predicted will occur and veterinary surgeons will be involved in discussing the impact of these changes.

As we increase the meat requirements of the global population then intensification of the dairy, beef, sheep and goat industries seems inevitable. This intensification will require that animals are kept in high standards of care and veterinary surgeons will be pivotal in helping this come about. It may be that new protein food sources may replace these traditional farm animals and change the look of farming. Fish farming already occurs with its intensification problems, prawns and other shell-fish are harvested; insects are a protein source in some nations. These may well change the relative desire for beef, sheep, poultry and pig. The overall impact on welfare of the farm animals is very difficult if not impossible to predict.

Advances in our ability to treat animals will allow us to cure animals that are currently difficult or impossible to treat. This change will allow us to improve the welfare of afflicted animals but it may be that this ability to treat will reduce the drive to prevent conditions and may lead to veterinary surgeons covering up a dysfunctional system. New treatments are usually expensive – although not always – but where they are it reduces the overall resources that can be spread to other animals. It is possible that renal transplantation, sophisticated surgical techniques and medical treatments that can only be speculated at now will be of immense benefit to an individual animal but could result in a reduced ability to improve the welfare of all animals.

Refinements in technology may be able to detect disease earlier and reduce the impact of disease. Improved diagnosis will improve the veterinary surgeon's ability to work with owners and will be invaluable in working with all aspects to detect and deal with issues in a timely manner.

10

VETERINARY SURGEONS AND POLITICS

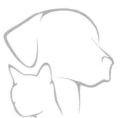

Veterinary surgeons are particularly involved in politics as a profession and appear to be one of the most organised groups when it comes to working with the legislature of countries and regions. Either on an individual level or as a grouping of like-minded professionals they will campaign to influence the legislation at any of the levels from local issues through to supra-national legislation and problems.

The professional organisations such as the British Veterinary Association and the American Veterinary Medical Association will work to represent their members to their respective governments, whether these are the devolved regions of the UK, the state legislatures in the USA, the Westminster parliament or the federal government in Washington, DC. In Europe there are associations that will represent members in their country to the national government and the European Parliament. The Federation of Veterinarians of Europe works to take a coordinated message to bodies such as the European Parliament from all of the veterinary organisations throughout Europe.

Other veterinary surgeons will work as individuals; they may work on issues that are close to their heart or particularly local (and may have nothing to do with the profession at all). Government veterinary surgeons may not be able to comment on the reasoning behind the decisions and policies that they have to implement but there is obviously a political dimension to the work.

WHY ARE VETS INVOLVED IN POLITICS?

There are many possible reasons that veterinary surgeons are so involved in politics as individuals and as a profession. Veterinary surgeons will have differing motivations to become involved in politics but there are some common reasons why they might become involved; particularly those involved in food production.

Food – and particularly food of an animal origin – is an emotive subject and encompasses welfare, environmental, human health and provenance issues. The production of food is not only important to consumers because of welfare issues and health but also because of the use of medications that may contaminate the food chain. Provenance of food is also considered important, as the horsemeat scandal in 2014 demonstrated. Ensuring that the regulation supports this in a proportionate and justifiable manner is a political issue and veterinary surgeons are involved in all of these issues.

Veterinary practices have traditionally been small businesses with a few veterinary surgeons and some support staff. Where there is a farming community that the practice serves then the farms have traditionally also been effectively small businesses. Supporting the farming community makes sense for the veterinary profession, as they are part of that community and derive their income from that community. They are well placed as a profession to comment on the issues that are raised because of their training in scientific matters combined with an understanding of the pressures on the farming community. Despite the fact that the veterinary profession is so closely involved in the farming industry, it is still widely regarded as an honest and impartial voice on most matters associated with agriculture. So veterinary surgeons become involved in political issues to support their business and the business of their clients but do so in a manner that is for the benefit of all, including the animals under their care and the consumers that will be purchasing the products.

As a veterinary student there is a culture of wider involvement in issues beyond the personal that is inculcated during the training. This is partly due to the lecturers themselves being asked to comment on issues because of their high degree of expertise. Their contribution to the political debate will inevitably leak through to students in lectures or by the media discussions involving the university staff. The veterinary student voice is also listened to through the Association of Veterinary Students in the UK, or the Student American Veterinary Medical Association. Both of these organisations respect the voice of their student members as the future of the profession and Australia, New Zealand and other countries have similar organisations that gather and publicise the opinion of the student body. So once a veterinary student has graduated, they are already steeped in a culture of getting involved beyond the day-to-day job.

The decision to study veterinary medicine is frequently motivated by the chance to work with animals but another important motivation is a desire to improve the lot of others through improving the wild environment, improving the nutrition of people in impoverished areas or many other reasons more specific to the veterinary surgeon concerned. The desire and motivation to change the world even in a small manner requires understanding of the politics of a situation and the wider the context of the intervention, the more important the politics associated with the attempt to make improvements in areas may be.

Other professions impact on veterinary medicine and negotiation between the various professionals sometimes emerges into politics as regulations are developed. Probably the most current example of this is the use of antibiotics in farm animals, due to the suspicion that the use of some classes of antibiotics as treatments for bacterial diseases of farm livestock may lead to resistance in bacteria it has been proposed that the use of many types of antibiotic is reduced. Those veterinary surgeons involved in the discussion with politicians are seeking to ensure that the regulations that are developed are proportionate and reasonable as well as achieving the aim of preserving the antibiotic types as effective medication for the humans and animals that need it. Non-stun slaughter is another area where intense political discussion has taken place (and will likely continue) in order to again produce regulations that are proportionate and reasonable.

As outlined there are many reasons for engaging in political activity and it is probably not surprising that the veterinary surgeons working with farm animals are most involved, but others are also involved and there may be as many motivations as there are veterinary surgeons. Political activity can take many forms; signing a petition can be a way of influencing the development of regulations or policies.

Internet forums are used by many organisations (not just veterinary organisations) and the views of the profession are often gathered in this way.

Consultations are documents produced by government departments to gather the views of interested stakeholders (individuals or organisations that may have an interest or be affected by the subject being discussed). These views are gathered through the forums and committees and individuals may write responses to the consultations individually. Most governments in all countries have similar processes, although the name and detail of the presentation of the document and way the response is submitted may differ.

Most organisations will have a committee structure to ensure that the members are represented accurately and well. These may well represent the view of the organisation through written evidence to government committees. In addition, the chair of the committee may give oral evidence to the government.

Politics is a primary function of the government and veterinary surgeons are employed by the government to work in this area. Most countries have a head veterinary surgeon – the chief veterinary officer – who is responsible for developing, applying and monitoring governmental policy regarding animal health and welfare. They will be supported by other vets who may have more expertise in specific areas, who will assist in developing policies and responding to developing situations such as notifiable disease outbreaks. They may also request advice from members of the profession that are noted for their skills and knowledge in a relevant area. Those veterinary surgeons working in government service may have to be careful when making comments as they may be taken as the official government policy.

NOTABLE VETERINARY SURGEONS IN POLITICS

There have been many veterinary surgeons that have gone into politics as a progression of their career. They have been regional representatives such as members of parliament in Australia and Canada. They have been in the House of Representatives and Senate in the USA.

In the UK, the political system also has two different bodies that decide laws, the House of Commons and the House of Lords and two veterinary surgeons have been admitted to the House of Lords on the merit of their work.

Lord Soulsby

Lord Soulsby was the first veterinary surgeon admitted to the House of Lords. His peerage – the Lord Soulsby of Swaffham Prior – was created in 1990 following a career in veterinary medicine that took him from his graduation at Edinburgh to time at Bristol, Philadelphia and Cambridge University. His written output amounts to 14 books and more than 200 articles covering many aspects of veterinary medicine. His work at the House of Lords has seen him contributing to the work on the Science and Technology Committee and the Committee on Animals in Scientific Procedures. His policy interests are science technology, agriculture and food production alongside education and international affairs. This is all alongside chairing the Companion Animal Welfare Council, the Pet Advisory Council and the Windward Islands Research and Education Foundation.

Lord Trees

The second veterinary surgeon to be admitted to the House of Lords was Professor Alexander Trees. Coincidentally he also graduated, like Lord Soulsby, from the University of Edinburgh.

He was created as Baron Trees, of the Ross in Perth and Kinross in 2012. Lord Trees sits on committees covering agriculture, fisheries and energy and the environment. His policy areas cover veterinary and tropical medicine as well as many others.

Professor Christianne Glossop

Although veterinary surgeons that work for the government are restrained by the policies of the government of the day, some have made great strides for the animals in their jurisdiction. Professor Christianne Glossop is just such an individual. A graduate of the Royal Veterinary College as an undergraduate and with a PhD in cattle fertility, she was appointed as the first chief veterinary officer of Wales in 2005. Her tenure in this post has seen the development of progressive and forward-thinking strategies in combatting bovine TB in Wales. This has included providing a better testing framework and integrating the private veterinary surgeon working for the farmer into the control of the disease much more effectively. Her leadership within Wales has seen the closer partnership with all of the people and organisations involved in animal health and welfare and her tenure may see the establishment of a new veterinary course within Wales; an achievement that all veterinary surgeons would be proud to have seen within their career.

VETERINARY SURGEONS IN POLITICS

The veterinary profession is well organised and represented as a political organisation. The various groups that form around an identity as a veterinary surgeon – such as the AVMA, the AVA or the BVA – and those that have a narrower specialisation do an impressive job of representing the view of the members and of producing a balanced view on many subjects. It is a credit to the profession that throughout the world the views expressed by these organisations and individual veterinary surgeons is considered as fair and trustworthy. Hopefully this will continue into the future.

11

VETERINARY SURGEONS IN SCIENCE

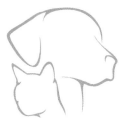

KEY POINTS

- All veterinary surgeons are trained scientists.

- The route through a PhD is common for many veterinary surgeons.

- Many have contributed to the advancement of many areas of science.

- Findings are presented in papers that allow everyone to assess the findings and check them.

All veterinary surgeons are involved in science and are educated in science throughout their training. Outside the clinical career path there are a number of veterinary surgeons that will undertake a complete career working in research.

The exposure of a veterinary student to conducting research starts with the requirement of many courses for at least one research project. Some university courses will require more than one. These research projects can range in scope from working in a laboratory on a detailed examination of a specific molecule or pathway through to the effect of interventions on whole populations. Most undergraduate research projects will be based on work that established research teams in the university are already working on. This has the advantage of allowing the student to benefit from the experience embedded within the research team. Depending on the academic regulations then it is possible that the student will be expected to complete one project on their own.

For those that have an increased interest then intercalating within the undergraduate course is an option. For those attending Cambridge University, this is a compulsory part of the course but all universities in the UK offer this as an option. Intercalating involves the student pausing in the veterinary training that they are involved in. They will then spend a year studying a specific area in greater detail. These can be related to the veterinary career – such as pathology – but increasingly these courses are aimed at teaching a one-health viewpoint and the course may be studied with medical students. A few students will undertake a course for that year that is completely different from the scientific veterinary course.

There are many reasons for intercalating. It may be that the student wishes to look at the subject in more detail, it may allow a greater interest in an area to be developed. More prosaically, the intercalation may be beneficial to the student as the extra qualification can be an advantage over others who do not have an intercalated degree. Of course the type and grade achieved in the intercalated degree may also be important in differentiating between candidates for research careers or possibly other career options.

ROUTE TO A SCIENTIFIC CAREER

Once the veterinary degree has been obtained then the graduate may wish to continue their studies at a more advanced level. Universities in the United States will offer combined DVM/PhD programmes as the entrance requirements will mean that the students will have the undergraduate degree already but usually the PhD will be obtained after the veterinary degree. The PhD is the usual prerequisite for embarking on a research career. The term PhD is used to denote that the holder is a doctor of philosophy and there are a number of variants to the letters that those who hold this qualification can use. Holders have undertaken a three-year research-based training programme and will have written a thesis based on the research undertaken during that time. A thesis is a text explaining the importance of the research undertaken and giving the results of that work. The written work of the student is usually significant in terms of word count as well, with 100,000 words being typical. An alternative to the thesis submission is to be required to submit a number of articles (frequently referred to as papers) to a journal and have them published for all who may be interested in the results. The student will then typically be asked to defend the thesis by discussing the thesis with a group (two or more) of experts in the field of study that the thesis covers. This discussion will explore the students' depth of knowledge of the subject area to ensure that there is an ability to place the work done by the student into context when the whole of the knowledge gained by the scientific community on that subject. The limitations of the work will also be explored in detail both to allow the student to correct the work in subsequent rewrites and to ensure the student understands the limitations of the work carried out.

The outcome of the defence of the student's thesis will result in a pass (allowing the student to progress forward to other careers), a fail (meaning that the student cannot continue) or a rewrite to correct major or minor flaws may be required by the examining committee after which the PhD will be awarded.

Throughout the studies to complete a PhD, the student will have at least one or two supervisors to help and guide the programme. These will usually be the principal investigator of a research programme that has managed to get funds for teaching PhD students and training new researchers.

While the measure of success for a veterinary surgeon in clinical veterinary practice might be the successful treatment of the animal or group of animals, when the veterinary surgeon is working in a research environment, the criteria of success is different. Research is reported to other people through papers and presentations at conferences.

WHAT IS A PAPER?

In order to report the findings of any research project, the results are reported in journals (magazines) that specialize in publishing these reports of the research in a specific area. These reports have a specific structure that has developed over years and consists of an abstract, introduction, materials and methods section and a final discussion section.

The abstract summarises the key points in the paper and is useful in allowing the reader to decide whether it is of interest to them. This is followed by the introduction, which outlines why the research was done and why it may be important to answer the question posed and this question will usually be made explicit in this section. Materials and methods are outlined in the next section in a faithful and accurate description of the techniques carried out and the supplies used in order to carry out the research.

The results section is probably the most important section in any paper. It sets out the findings in tables, pictures and any other format that the author thinks is required to demonstrate the findings in a clear manner. This is done without the author's interpretation of the data and findings, and the discussion section allows the author to provide their interpretation of the data and place into the context of the wider literature as the author sees it. The results section is therefore probably one of the most important sections, as this allows the author to justify their arguments and the reader to decide whether the interpretation is valid for themselves. However, the discussion section allows the authors to interpret the data and place it in what they perceive to be the appropriate context.

How many of these are produced by an individual researcher is variable. There is no doubt that some researchers are extremely productive and will produce many pieces of work in a year while others will be lucky to produce one. In any case, it is true that career satisfaction here is gained in a different way to the veterinary surgeon working in clinical practice. Those working in either field will find satisfaction in whatever career they chose but the way these are delivered will be different.

Once the manuscript is prepared to the authors' satisfaction then the next step is to select and submit to the journal.

PEER REVIEW

Once the journal receives a submitted article, it starts a process that is in place to provide some level of quality assurance. This is the peer review process and it will make sure that there are at least no major errors of fact, writing or interpretation. It is impossible to catch all of them and it is very difficult to catch deliberate fraud at this point.

All information is subject to this limitation, it depends critically on the honesty and integrity of the workers who carry out the research. Integrity of research is an area that will develop, as will the ways in which research is disseminated to the members of the profession. Currently the access is through peer-reviewed journals that the reader subscribes to, either directly or through their employers. Much research is paid for through general taxation. Open access and review through subscriber comments may become more common in order to ensure that the government gets more value for money for the research that it pays for.

EVIDENCE-BASED MEDICINE

Research is the cornerstone of evidence-based veterinary medicine (EBVM). This is a way of thinking that has recently been codified to help clinicians make the best decisions for their clients. Good quality research underpins this decision making process. EBVM starts by clarifying the question that the clinician is asking themselves to make it relevant to their situation. The clinician must be able to decide on the quality of the research presented for themselves. Not all research is of the same quality, or appropriate for the question that the clinician is interested in. A skill is to decide how much weight to place on any given piece of research.

Even when a single piece of research is carried out to the highest of standards then the results are not definitively true. Each result is associated with a p-value. This is a statement of its statistical significance. Interpretation of the p- value is complex and frequently confused but a simplified explanation is that the lower the p-value the lower the chance of getting a result demonstrating a positive result in a lower number of repeated studies. For example if we have a p-value of 0.05 and our hypothesis is wrong then if we ran 100 studies, 95 would show no difference, which would be correct, and five studies that would show a difference, which would not reflect the true situation. The only way to determine whether we have a true difference in our research question or we have an unusual study sample is replication of the research by multiple groups.

SIGNIFICANT VETERINARY SCIENTISTS

There are many veterinary surgeons that are involved in science. The most well-known prize awarded to scientists of any background is a Nobel Prize. Only one veterinary surgeon has (to date) won a Nobel Prize – Peter Charles Doherty. He is an Australian who studied veterinary medicine at the University of Queensland and got his PhD at the University of Edinburgh. The research that won Dr Doherty his Nobel Prize was carried out at the John Curtin School of Medical Research in Canberra alongside a colleague Rolf Zinkernagel. They carried out work to define the mechanics of defence against viral infection. They demonstrated the requirement for the major histocompatibility complex in recognizing that a virus has infected a cell and initiating protective responses.

Although winning prizes is probably not a major motivation to veterinary surgeons, many have contributed to our understanding of the world. There are thousands working in universities and research establishments all around the world. Throughout the history of the profession, some veterinary surgeons have come to the attention of the public.

Bernhard Bang

Brucellosis is an important disease of both people and animals and has been known as a disease since antiquity particularly by the people of the Mediterranean. British medical officers were the first to write about the disease as Malta fever and Bernhard Bang quickly realized that a bacteria – *Brucella abortus* – was responsible for the clinical signs seen in Malta fever or undulant fever.

Sir Arnold Theiler

Theileriosis is a disease of animals that is caused by single-celled parasites and is found in Africa. Arnold Theiler was instrumental in defining the disease and once the causative agent was identified it was named in his honour as *Theileria Parva*. He also identified the similarly named Theiler's disease, a liver inflammation that he identified as being associated with the treatment of horses with a medicine derived from other horses such as antitoxins. A virus of the pegivirus genus has recently been associated with this disease. Sir Arnold was also instrumental in setting up veterinary research and teaching in Southern Africa.

James Alexander Thompson

A graduate of the DVM programme at the University of Pennsylvania and a molecular biologist, James Alexander Thompson was the first scientist to derive and grow human embryonic stem cells. This allowed research into many areas of human development, transplantation and drug development.

Professor Brian Derek Perry

It is not only the lab-based sciences that attract the attention of veterinary surgeons to look deeper and try and get a better understanding of a specific field. Some are interested in the interaction of animals, people and disease in the field. Professor Perry has contributed to the understanding of veterinary epidemiology and economics. This has led to work in developing disease and research priorities for countries in Africa, and South America focusing on tropical diseases. This has led to work on poverty reduction. This work has allowed for the best use of resources to combat the most important diseases.

Jean-Marie Camille Guérin

Born in France, Jean-Marie Camille Guérin developed the BCG vaccine (bacillus Calmette-Geurin) by treating (attenuating) the bacterium mycobacterium bovis that causes bovine TB. They grew the bacterium over 230 generations at the Institute Pasteur de Lille. This vaccine is still an important tool in the control of human TB in areas where the disease is still common.

Robert Royston Amos Coombs

The Coombs test is used in human medicine to test for autoimmune haemolytic anaemia in its direct form and to detect rhesus positive antibodies in pregnant women and to determine the suitability of blood transfusions. This test has allowed countless safe transfusions to take place.

Veterinary surgeons in research will have many reasons for undertaking research. What will not appear is a desire for a large salary. Chapter 7 goes into detail about the salary expectations of the career in comparison to the rest of the profession and the general population.

A passion for a specific subject is a frequent reason that the individual will choose the career path and some will be able to combine this with clinical work either due to their area of interest involving clinical patients or they continue the clinical work in parallel with their research work. The contribution that veterinary surgeons make to human and animal health cannot be understated and the few described in this chapter are just examples of the many that work tirelessly in laboratories, on farms and in clinics, interviewing clients producing work to improve animal health. Even those who do come to the attention of the general public for their work will be building on the work carried out by colleagues both veterinary and non-veterinary.

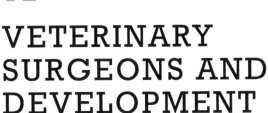

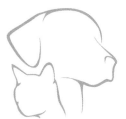

12

VETERINARY SURGEONS AND DEVELOPMENT

KEY POINTS

- Veterinary surgeons can contribute to the health and feeding of populations that are in need.

- Frequently veterinary surgeons are involved in training local people in skills that they don't have rather than treating animals directly.

- The variety of organisations means that every need is covered.

INTRODUCTION

Veterinary surgeons at all stages of their career express an interest in working abroad and helping local communities in Africa, Asia and South America in the many developing countries. The time that veterinary surgeons spend in countries that are termed 'developing' is varied, as are their motivations for being there and the activities they will take part in. The effect they have is hopefully positive but history of interference in this area is frequented with efforts that have gone astray.

WHAT DO WE MEAN?

Working in development generally refers to those who work in those countries that are defined by criteria that suggest there is an increased level of absolute and relative poverty. These definitions are vague, not universally accepted and may not accurately reflect the general perception of a developing country or the actual state of affairs in the whole country. A simple definition of these countries might be a lowered life expectancy, an increased infant mortality and reduced income for its inhabitants. These characteristics are likely to fit any countries that veterinary surgeons might be motivated to work in.

It is important for those from Europe, the USA, Canada, Australia and New Zealand to understand that these developing countries are not totally without locally trained veterinary surgeons, but there may be problems with the infrastructure such as access to resources for training, lack of ability to get the veterinary surgeons to the animals due to poor transport, poor access to diagnostic laboratories and lack of access to medicines through poor resources or a poor cold chain damaging or destroying the efficacy of medicines and in particular vaccines. This veterinary medicine infrastructure problem of countries is something that the World Organisation for Animal Health (OIE) is particularly aware of and it has set up a programme to help produce a sustainable improvement in the veterinary services that are provided by the government of these countries. This means that the provision of veterinary services by foreign vets directly to local famers and animal owners may reduce the opportunities for employment and once the veterinary surgeon has moved away from the local area or country the skills and knowledge also move. Building an infrastructure that will be there in the long term should be the goal of development agencies.

Animals are important parts of the gross domestic product of any country, but developing countries probably rely on animals more than those countries that are developed. Animals are important in food production as food items (meat, milk and eggs) and as power to produce crops in areas where tractors are too expensive or unable to cope with terrain. Locally trained veterinary surgeons are sometimes available but the infrastructure to support them may not be available. Colleagues from other countries are potentially valuable in improving the situation for these local vets and the communities that they work in.

Veterinary surgeons can be involved in training the local farmers, veterinary surgeons or paravets (local people who work with the local livestock population and provide simple routine care such as parasite control). This is an extremely valuable contribution to the care of animals in the rural communities that these individuals generally work in.

Animals are also a potential cause of zoonotic (animal to man transmission) disease and these are increasingly important in developing countries as there are more in the surrounding environment; in addition, the human health infrastructure may be under as much pressure as the veterinary one. If the work of veterinary surgeons can reduce the risk of zoonotic diseases to the people of the country then this will improve. Working to ensure that farm animals are healthy and disease-free can do this. The food chain can be protected, with veterinary surgeons working to ensure that – with the resources available to the local population – the risks from eating contaminated food are reduced as much as possible. This will then reduce the pressure on hospitals and medical clinics.

Feral and wild animals are another source of infection for humans and veterinary surgeons will work to reduce the number of adverse interactions and the risks associated with these interactions. Education of the population can lead to a reduction of animal attacks, as local attitudes to animals can be changed. This can lead to a reduction of attacks on people and livestock, which has the additional advantage of a reduction in resentment of local wildlife. Feral dogs – domesticated dogs that have been abandoned and are now living wild – are found throughout the world and many veterinary surgeons will become involved in neutering and vaccinating these animals. Neutering will reduce the breeding population and, over time, the numbers of animals that can pose a risk. Vaccination for rabies can reduce the number of animals that can carry the disease and infect people following an attack or bite. These interventions will also make a positive impact on the health and welfare of the animal population as repeat breeding will increase the number of animals putting pressure on the food resources (generally rubbish from homes and businesses). This increasing pool of animals will also maintain a virus, such as rabies, that can infect humans. Vaccination will reduce the pool of susceptible animals and protect both the human and wildlife population.

NEW AND EMERGING DISEASES

There are many diseases that are found in the tropical countries that are able to infect people through animals such as rabies, trypanosomiasis (sleeping sickness) and many others, but it is considered that many of the new and as yet unknown zoonotic diseases will come from the interaction of humans and wildlife in tropical countries. As these countries are more likely to be developing and have the medical (veterinary and human) infrastructure that is under massive pressure, then disease is likely to spread much more quickly. A particularly tragic example of this is the Ebola outbreak of 2014. The first disease associated with filoviruses (the family of viruses that Ebola belongs to) was first identified through infection of laboratory workers, but Ebola was identified in 1976 following outbreaks in Zaire and Sudan. This disease kept recurring in the intervening period and the latest outbreak has tragically killed 9,019 people and infected 22,560 people (these figures include suspected as well as confirmed cases). The work of many people helped to control this outbreak but the risks are clear and should be kept in mind.

WHAT ARE VETERINARY SURGEONS' MOTIVATIONS FOR GETTING INVOLVED?

As with the political issues that veterinary surgeons might be involved with, there are many underlying reasons why a veterinary surgeon might be involved in working in the developing world. At the university once again there is an emphasis on working to improve the lot of others and this can be animals directly or the improvement of the life of people through the better use and productivity of animals. Another reason might be a fascination with the subjects that are more directly involved in developing countries, such as parasite diseases that are found in these areas.

Religious motivations may also be important in motivating veterinary surgeons to work in developing areas, as missionary work may be required or a desire of the individual.

PERSONAL HEALTH AND SAFETY

Unlike when doctors work in developing countries, veterinary surgeons are not commonly involved in the primary response to disasters or conflicts. This reduces the danger but does not remove it completely. A suitable vaccination programme for anyone travelling should be completed, and measures to protect health (mosquito nets, for example) should be remembered. Insurance is a wise investment.

Crime can be a problem in any country but normal precautions should suffice. Attitudes may differ in many countries and behaviour should be adjusted accordingly, blending in will minimise the chances of problems and will probably improve the experience anyway.

SOME ISSUES ABOUT CHARITABLE PROJECTS

There are many reasons to get involved in the work to improve animal health and welfare in developing countries and veterinary surgeons can get involved at any stage of their career – from the undergraduate stage to highly experienced researchers and clinicians. Choosing a project that you are passionate about is a good first step, as the resources are likely to be limited and a highly motivated member of the team may bring a fresh way to use these limited resources effectively. If nothing else, the energy of a motivated individual may bring a new energy and enthusiasm to the team.

Understanding the project is another recommended prerequisite and this involves not just the technical aspects of the project but also having some appreciation of the culture of the country that the project is based in. Although the chance to experience a new culture and learn about the country and people is one of the reasons why these experiences are sometimes taken on, it will increase the chance of a positive experience if there is a basic appreciation and sympathy of the local sensitivities. This is sometimes interpreted that the local mores should have significance over the welfare needs of the animal concerned. The balance needs to be determined for each situation, remembering the priorities and resources available to the local communities. When the choice is between treating a child and dealing with a sick animal, the child is always going to take priority.

The projects in developing countries are going to have local employees and these people should be treated fairly. This can be as simple as referring to them by the appropriate name and respecting their position within their society. This may be a problem for some as it may mean working with people who have social views that are antithetical to theirs. This is a difficult area but if the project is to be successful then it will need to be considered.

Many veterinary surgeons will go across and conduct training courses for livestock farmers. Training of people in skills is a useful and sustainable way forward but it must be careful that the local veterinary surgeons do not appear to be less valuable or are undermined. In some areas of this work, the public face of many initiatives is always a local person and the foreign team members are support and provide specialist skills and training – training the trainers.

The project may be counterproductive; there are certainly some concerns about the sending of animals to people in the developing world in order to increase the food production. Done well, this is a great initiative but the recipient has to be able to work with these animals and have appropriate support. Although volunteers are unlikely to be in a position to change a project, veterinary surgeons may work for charities that operate in these countries and consideration should be given to the full and wider impact of any interventions.

It would appear that volunteering and working in development projects is difficult and potentially ineffective, but careful consideration of the project by those working on it should avoid these. It is a testament to the skills of the veterinary profession that these issues are avoided.

ANIMAL-BASED DEVELOPMENT ORGANISATIONS

There are many organisations working to support the people of the developing world in many ways, including many aspects of animal use, health and welfare. Some of the organisations will be familiar as they also work in Europe, Northern America, Australia and New Zealand, such as the Donkey Sanctuary, which works to protect the welfare of donkeys and mules throughout the world. Donkeys and mules are commonly used in agriculture, providing power and transporting people and goods. The use of these animals does contribute to the health and welfare of the people in many areas but the animals may not be well cared for. This may be for the reasons indicated above, such as lack of resources or expertise. This organisation provides veterinary services to the animals and educates the owners about appropriate care of these animals. This education and the work that is carried out are underpinned by research that the sanctuary has commissioned.

Another organisation that works with donkeys due to their utility to the local population as well as desire to improve the life of these undervalued animals is SPANA. All working animals are cared for at SPANA veterinary clinics throughout the world. These clinics are mobile and travel huge distances to reach animals that require care. SPANA will also provide emergency interventions where required. However, these programmes are only part of the solution and must be combined with education to build knowledge and promote responsible behaviour and empathy with an aim to build a populace with an attitude to animals that is friendly to the welfare of the animals.

The Brooke is another charity that works to provide veterinary care, education and training that is relevant to the animals and people of the developing world. This is underpinned by research that is another aspect of the charity's work. The Brooke is also involved in working with the governments and policymakers of various countries to assist with the development of an appropriate infrastructure. A key component is the transfer of the concept of the Five Freedoms to the developed world and developing welfare measurement techniques and applying them to check whether any interventions are successful. Building an infrastructure is, as already indicated, an important part of working in the development work.

Vétérinaires Sans Frontières (VSF) is a charity based in Belgium that works to build the network of private practices in rural areas, as well as provide support for these and for the authorities with responsibility for animals. Trade in animals is also important in improving the life of people in developing countries and VSF works to support the trade of animals through assisting in getting products to market and assisting in providing small loans to local people to allow them to make investments that will provide for their families in the future. In the areas where VSF works, pasture and water may be scarce. It is important to protect these resources and VSF will work with the communities to achieve this, alongside working with the local populations to protect the natural environment. As with the other charities, VSF will provide education that will allow the people to develop their own solutions to the problems they face on a day-to-day basis. Allowing the local population to develop their own solutions by providing the knowledge that allows this is an important aspect of this whole area and Vetaid Kenya is a charity that developed from an older charity and now consists of local Kenyan workers (veterinary surgeons and animal health workers) and has an association with the Royal Veterinary College (RVC) in London, which allows this charity access to the latest information to take back to Kenya and further develop their response to emergencies. Like many of these organisations, Vetaid Kenya does not work in isolation and alongside its partnership with the RVC it works with other partners such as GALVMED, which works to build the all-important infrastructure in the countries it has determined are in need of support. The supply of money or information is one aspect of the work that occurs but money can potentially be diverted from those who need it most. Women, for example, are often thought to be disproportionately affected by poverty but supplying animals may avoid this issue. One organisation that does this is Send a Cow. Alongside the supply of livestock, it provides training in keeping livestock and farming those livestock to try and improve the ability of the local people to generate food and income.

The armed forces of many countries have a veterinary component, such as the British Royal Army Veterinary Corps, the US Army Veterinary Corps, the Australian Army Veterinary Corps or any of the other countries with such organisations. These corps and units are frequently used in disaster relief to alleviate the immediate problems. Additionally as part of deployments, the men and women of these units will work with local populations to bring about an improvement in the production and welfare of the animals in the country.

Livestock have a vital role in feeding the population of any country but are particularly important in countries where the country as a whole cannot compete in the international market to import food. Livestock are not the only animals that require care and suffer from the lack of veterinary services with the country. Dogs, cats and wildlife also require care. As with livestock, charitable organisations have been set up to fill this need. One is Vets Beyond Borders, which provides voluntary veterinary surgeons to work on population control through neutering animals and controlling rabies through vaccination. Training of local veterinary surgeons is also undertaken and is part of building an infrastructure that can allow the development of stray dog policies that are more welfare friendly.

The Worldwide Veterinary Service (WVS) fulfils a similar role in providing vaccination neutering and training. The WVS has vaccinated for both rabies as a human health problem and distemper to protect the dogs from disease outbreaks. WVS also responds to disasters and emergencies whether they occur in the developing world or not.

These charities provide valuable assistance to the people of the developing world and demonstrate the value of veterinary input into human health and the professions' contribution to the world and are all deserving of the profession's backing, whether that is time or financial support.

13
FUTURE
SCANNING

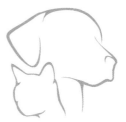

Predicting the future is fraught with difficulty and many people have embarrassed themselves trying. The rate of change is incredible in many fields of human endeavour and veterinary medicine is no different, and changes in other areas will impact on the future career of students entering the profession so some indication of the future direction should be given to the potential candidates. Although it is difficult to accurately predict what will happen – particularly over the next five years, ten years or longer timescale – but it has to be done at many levels in order to make plans. Governments in particular will do so in order to assign resources, universities will do so to produce graduates that are equipped for their futures and students will do so for the same reasons.

In the UK there are a total of seven veterinary schools that a student who wishes to become a veterinary surgeon can apply to. Five have been in existence for decades, two have opened up in the past ten years – Nottingham and Surrey universities. This increases the number of places available to the prospective student. Alongside the opening of these university courses, the other courses are increasing the intake of students per year and this increase within schools may well increase the number of students more than the opening of new courses, although the latter attracts more interest from the media and the veterinary profession. Nottingham and Surrey may not be the only universities to open courses, as other universities seem to be contemplating doing so too. Aberystwyth has been open about its ambitions in this direction and rumours abound about other universities also having similar plans. The choice of veterinary courses available to the students in the UK may increase due to changes in the application process. UCAS – the organisation that manages this process for all the UK students who wish to go to university – has started to work with universities in the rest of Europe. This is likely to increase the number of places available for the students in the UK to apply to. Obviously this will require that the students applying will have appropriate language skills but over time the most plausible result of this change is the gradual increase in the number of veterinary students competing for places in European courses. These may then return home and this will put further pressure on extra-mural studies, jobs and salary levels.

The impact on the applicants is obviously to increase the opportunities for joining a course. Changes in the requirements for the academic and extracurricular activities are probably not going to become less stringent unless the popularity of the profession as a whole somehow decreases. The number of applicants per year is currently 8–10 per place available. The chances of enough places becoming available to make a difference to this ratio are not high.

There is a school of thought within the profession that the type of student being recruited is not displaying the aptitude that is desired on qualification. This is partially addressed by the BMAT that is required by many of the UK universities but alternative selection procedures may be used; with many processes success is defined in large parts by ensuring that it operates on the best components. In the case of education, it is the students themselves that are responsible for the success. Passing the examinations is one measure but another is the ability to perform successfully as a qualified veterinary surgeon. Universities like to have a reputation for success and if the weight moves from success at the qualification level to success in the career then they will be looking for ways of determining likely success as early as possible through the selection process. How this will be carried out may be through observation of key characteristics or ways of interacting with people or animals.

The UK is not the only country where numbers of courses are increasing; the US had two new veterinary courses that were seeking accreditation in 2014 (Midwestern in Arizona and Lincoln Memorial in Tennessee). As with the situation in the UK, the number of courses in the US will probably increase. There is a slow growth as regards the number of places within the existing veterinary schools in the USA as well.

This increase in student numbers that appears to be happening all over the world has been associated with a reduction in the staff-to-student ratio. This increase of students per member of staff is a problem across the world as student numbers increase in each college. This puts pressure on the resources and student interaction with the subject experts, particularly in the clinical years. This pressure may change the type of person who is willing to train veterinary students. Traditionally the instructors have also been heavily involved in the research being carried out in the university. Time pressure due to the time invested in student teaching of larger numbers (this includes lesson preparation, exam marking, feedback, etc.) may require changes in the methods of delivery. Some universities have made the decision to employ some vets as purely educators. This may bring about the creation of veterinary surgeons that are primarily educators. Lecturers with this single focus, professional educators, may provide a better service as trainers. Another view may be that this will reduce access for veterinary undergraduates to the new research and thinking and will reduce the quality overall. As with many things, a balance between the two views will probably provide an optimum solution.

The cost of undertaking a veterinary course is subject to many pressures. The UK government pays for the undergraduate training of students from the UK but requires a contribution in the form of student fees. The level that this is set at is a matter of government policy. The effect on student fees will depend on the overall economy and maintaining a sustainable education in the light of the country's overall economic performance. Further increase cannot be ruled out, obviously.

Extra-mural studies (EMS) are carried out in the United Kingdom but are not a requirement for other countries. The increase of student numbers in the UK – whether that is through the opening of new veterinary schools or the increase in numbers at the school – has led to fears among the profession that this will increase the pressure on the practices in the UK that are willing to host students. The concern is that there will not be enough EMS placements available for students – although this might be over-exaggerating the issue, as there are plenty of willing placements that currently have few, if any, enquiries. The popular places will have many more applications than they can handle irrespective of the total number of students studying veterinary medicine. The delivery of EMS may have to be more carefully thought out and organised, with perhaps some form of centralised booking, as is carried out in some larger practice groups. Training of the veterinary practices and veterinary surgeons that deliver EMS may be desirable in order to improve the training that is given to undergraduates. This will increase the quality of the experience that the student based in the practice will gain; the universities may start to accredit practices and only permit their students to attend host practices in a manner reminiscent of the Bristol Foster practices. Or the structure of EMS may well change – at the time of writing, the RCVS is loosening the requirement for abattoir placements if the university can provide a sufficient replacement within the course. This may provide a model that can alter the requirements for EMS, or at least the composition. It would be disappointing if this were to be used to reduce or remove the EMS component of the veterinary course in the UK, as it is a valuable addition to the training of students by increasing the case exposure.

This change in EMS if it occurs will reflect the course structure and any changes that are made. Some European colleges have a specialisation during the undergraduate career and the training equips the graduates to deal with one broad class of animals, such as farm animals. Currently the UK, US, Australia and New Zealand will produce vets who are in principle capable of dealing with any species. There is a discussion whether this is sustainable and the volume of factual knowledge required of the students makes it very difficult to ensure that all students have the required knowledge. It would be a disappointing change to the training of veterinary students if the range of species dealt with were to be limited. Anecdotally there are many veterinary students that have qualified with a specific career path in mind who then change careers entirely. Additionally there are areas even in the UK where specialised veterinary surgeons are uneconomic due to population density. The ability to work with any species may be a valuable asset to the societies that live in these areas. What is required is evidence to determine how often career changes from livestock to equine to companion animal in any direction occur. This will gauge the impact of a change to pre-graduation specialisation (tracking in a specific species mix) on the future undergraduates.

The undergraduate curriculum of many veterinary courses has increasingly made claims to a 'one health' perspective. 'One health' is a mind-set regarding the optimal health of humans and animals. It posits that the challenges to human health will come from the interaction between animals and humans and the solutions to these problems will come from studying the common areas between animals and humans. Advances will come from interdisciplinary research, using animals as surveillance for human health risks such as contamination of food sources in the developing world. Increasing food production through better management and prevention strategies that veterinary surgeons are well trained in will also help the health of the local populations. As this 'one health' model is seen as benefiting the human population, it attracts strong funding and will be attractive to the universities that compete for research funds. It will depend on the research priorities of the veterinary universities whether they will compete for comparative or translational research funding, or epidemiology or surveillance research. Probably not surprisingly, the veterinary colleges and veterinary surgeons seem to have taken this thought process further than other disciplines such as the medical profession and hopefully the profession delivers the results that are hoped for by increasing the awareness of future graduates of their potential impact on the global human health situation.

The original veterinary profession was purely a clinical course but as a direct result of the demand from the customers (employers and graduates) the students are now being introduced to business concepts such as managing staff, personal and business finance and employment legislation. This trend is not going to reverse and where it may currently appear as an optional part of a veterinary curriculum, it will soon move to a core component. What this change will displace on any given curriculum will be dependent on the opinion of the stakeholders involved.

The type of applicant has changed gradually over time and there are an increasing number of women in the profession. This trend is likely to continue and will result in more women in practice, research and all the areas where veterinary surgeons work. The salary surveys conducted over the years have highlighted a disparity between what is paid to male and female veterinary surgeons; this gap is closing and will soon disappear if the trends continue in this direction. This positive development must be compared to the possibility that those professions that are dominated by women are generally less well paid than professions that are male-dominated. What the impact will be on the salary that female veterinary surgeons attract in the future is a matter of conjecture. It is to be hoped that the society as a whole will change to ensure that gender pay discrimination will not be an issue.

A veterinary profession with a majority female membership will face other challenges apart from the salary. More veterinary surgeons will require a work pattern that will support a family; maternity leave will quite correctly have to be accommodated. This may require more short-term contracts to cover leave, alongside an increase in the number of part-time jobs and job sharing. Traditional veterinary practices as small businesses may change; the common thought is that women are less likely to want to take on the role of practice partners and would rather prioritise other parts of life. This may drive the further progression of corporate practices. Within the veterinary organisations there should be a change in the leadership, with more women taking presidential positions of groups such as the BVA, the AVMA, EAVE, the RCVS and all the others that represent the veterinary profession if these are not to be seen as unrepresentative of the profession.

This change to a female-dominated profession may pose a challenge to many older members of society, particularly in the farming community, as some perceive female veterinary surgeons as being less capable, sometimes despite personal experience to the contrary. It will take a long time to change the societal perception that authority and gravitas are necessarily linked to grey-haired older men. While perhaps unfair, the professionalism of the veterinary profession should be sufficient to deal with even the more recalcitrant members of society to the benefit of all.

Upon graduation, each student will require a job, prosaically in order to pay bills, pay off debts and feed themselves, and to provide the self-esteem associated with being a successful professional. The job profile of the veterinary profession is almost certainly going to change. Currently the average graduating student expects to find a full-time position in clinical practice. As the demographic changes, the number of full-time positions may reduce to be replaced by a larger part-time workforce. This change may counter the increase in the number of veterinary surgeons that are available to fill these positions. This is both from the increase in places on the veterinary courses worldwide and the influx of veterinary surgeons from other countries. This is a particular concern in the UK where European-trained veterinary surgeons are permitted to work in the UK as a result of its membership of the European Union. These veterinary surgeons may have less debt and may be able and willing to accept lower salaries and poorer working conditions, putting a downward pressure on both. Veterinary surgeons may also be working in different positions than is currently perceived as the job. Research may attract more graduates, depending on the economic climate and changes in the government and other funding bodies potentially releasing increased research funding, while the public health aspect of veterinary training may become more important as the number and type of jobs increase, with the protection of the food supply increasing in importance. Another change in the jobs available may be an increase in specialisation of clinical veterinary positions. The mixed practice position is increasingly rare and the number of cat-only, farm veterinary-only, equine-only and all the other species-specific veterinary surgeons will almost certainly increase. It is possible that this will reduce the number of positions and practices available. A specialist in, for example, dairy cattle may be able to service more farms (and will need to do so to be economically viable). The pig, poultry and fish specialist veterinary surgeons are probably at the end of this process.

There are currently a number of system specialist veterinary surgeons working in practice outside the university/academic world and an increase in these may be seen as private practices seek to find a marketable difference, offer enhanced services and protect their client base. This in turn will increase the requirement for continuing professional development (CPD) training that is of high quality and provides a marketable skill. The training will have to be by veterinary surgeons and some practices are beginning to exploit this market already. The increasing specialisation will fragment the job market and provide more positions but those positions may be reduced in hours and will certainly involve contact with a reduced range of species.

The price of treatment associated with a profession that is increasingly specialised will increase. This price paid for this treatment reflects the increased training and increased equipment requirements, and as interventions become more sophisticated the medications will inevitably cost more. This increase may have changes that affect the animals being cared for. Insurance will be an increasingly important part of the veterinary business model. An increasing demand would be expected to tempt more companies into providing policies. This increase in a market that is already competitive may lead insurance companies into scrutinising bills more closely looking for value for money, effectiveness and efficient use of resources. This may be seen as an impingement on the clinical freedom of many veterinary surgeons but the growth of evidence-based medicine may leave fewer issues in terms of cost-effectiveness.

Evidence-based medicine it is hoped will continue to become more prominent. This will help veterinary surgeons determine the most effective treatments for their clients. Clinical governance will be aided as the veterinary surgeons can use the tools of evidence-based medicine to determine what procedures are performing poorly in their practice. By doing this as a profession, the practice of veterinary medicine should improve, with ineffective practices being weeded out.

The options available to veterinary surgeons when treating animals have increased enormously. There have been advances in imaging techniques, with digital X-rays becoming commonplace and more advanced techniques available. Sophisticated surgical techniques are available involving endoscopic techniques and implants with advanced materials. Medical interventions use increasingly sophisticated drugs such as angiotensin receptor blockers, interferons and erythropoietin. Transplants are offered in some cases and – although there are very real ethical concerns about this approach – it is almost certain that transplantation techniques will spread from renal transplantation in cats to other organs and species.

As more research is carried out on certain diseases we are increasingly able to prevent them. Vaccinations, already safe and effective, and the advice that we can use to prevent disease will become more refined as time goes on. In contrast to this increase in the sophistication of techniques, medications and advice, it is certain that practices that are currently used will be superseded by these newer techniques.

One aspect of evidence-based medicine is the knowledge of diseases that are present in any animal population and all governments require this information in order to develop animal health policy and research priorities. In the UK there has been a massive change in the delivery of this function, with the traditional veterinary laboratories being closed. Through conducting post-mortems and associated testing, these laboratories were able to build up a picture of the levels of disease in the country and detect novel diseases. The budget for this in the UK has been reduced and there are now concerns about the ability to deliver this information. The reduction in number of labs has left areas without cover due to the limitations of getting carcases to the locations of the new post-mortem expert providers. Alongside the changes to the post-mortem functions of the laboratories being altered (at least in the method of delivery) there may be more changes with an increase in active surveillance for specific diseases. There are projects that allow syndromic (looking for specific signs of illness) surveillance to be carried out within practice software. This type of approach might well expand but carries issues such as the accuracy of the data and client confidence in the security of their personal and business data. Other approaches using new technologies may also improve the accuracy and timeliness of data collection.

The future is likely to bring about new challenges in terms of the diseases and conditions that a veterinary surgeon will face in the future. New diseases will occur due to the increased interaction of humans and wildlife; hantavirus, Ebola virus and others will continue to emerge and challenge the human and animal health populations. This reflects a need for adequate surveillance in high-risk areas where new pathogens are likely to be found. These areas, such as rural Africa, South America and Asia, are where resources are limited and this increases the risk of missing the appearance of a disease until it has affected a large percentage of population. As air travel is a major part of the modern world, the spread can potentially be rapid. It will be slower in the animal population than in the human population, but avian influenza outbreaks still occur with surprising rapidity.

Diseases are not just caused by the presence of viruses, bacteria, parasites or fungi. Keeping the animal in a manner that does not meet the requirements that it needs or exposes it to novel risks can cause pathology or disease. Bovine spongiform encephalopathy (BSE) is one example of this novel disease that was thought to occur from a new management style (feeding meat and bone meal to dairy cattle) that carried with it a risk that was not understood. Currently in the UK there is discussion over the use of recycled manure solids. This is a method for reclaiming the fibre that is left in the faeces of cattle and using this material for bedding cattle in cubicles. The information is not there to determine whether this is safe in the UK (where weather conditions are different to other countries where it is used) and assessments are being carried out in order to make decisions about permitting the continued use in England and Scotland; Wales has not permitted the use of this material. However, even with a competent assessment there may be problems that are only seen when it is taken up by large numbers of farmers.

Companion animals are not immune to this issue either. There are always those animals new to the pet trade that find a fashionable niche; the list of new species viewed as pets increases constantly and can be influenced by children's films, books, celebrity endorsement and many other channels. Unfortunately many of these pets are sourced from the wild and the risk of these bringing novel diseases must be considered. Additionally the animals will have husbandry requirements that are poorly understood and may present to the veterinary surgeon with clinical signs that cannot be reliably linked to a disease process, as the underlying physiology is not well understood.

Changes in the keeping of traditional companion animals, such as dogs, cats and horses will bring new challenges and changes to the practice of veterinary medicine. These animals are living longer and the owners will ask for more extensive and sophisticated interventions and when these are no longer appropriate then the support around euthanasia will be expected to improve. As with people, these animals get the diseases and conditions that are associated with age such as cancer, arthritis and heart disease. Alongside these conditions, cognitive dysfunction is becoming of more interest with owners keen to preserve the animals as they were. Owners that are looking for this level of support are likely to have a significant emotional bond and look for enhanced help in trained counselling and grief support. It will have to be a practice decision whether this enhanced level of support is offered.

Even where the husbandry and physiological requirements of the animals under the care of the veterinary profession are understood, changes to the genetics of the animals may change the diseases seen. Breeding decisions may improve or reduce the immunity of animals, changes to the conformation of animals may produce breeding problems or uncover recessive and deleterious genes. There are many unknowns in this area and being responsive to the appearance of new conditions and using evidence-based medicine combined with a good surveillance of the diseases will allow the detection of issues. Breeding has in the past caused hip problems in dogs, breathing problems in short faced breeds, difficulty in giving birth due to wide heads in sheep and dogs and double muscling in cattle. These are being addressed in part but some breeds still have many flaws and many would be unrecognisable if the head shapes and other conformation problems were changed or removed.

The interventions available to the veterinary surgeon will not only increase but they will also decrease in some areas. Some medications will become unavailable to the profession. There are many reasons why this might occur and be occurring; a lot of media attention has been focused on the increase of antimicrobial resistance. The chief medical officer of England has suggested that the loss of antimicrobials is one of the most important dangers facing humanity. In order to address the rise of antimicrobial resistance, the US government has budgeted $1.2 billion to programmes that propose to address this. Many antibiotics have been used for a long period of time and resistance has developed among the bacteria found infecting animals; these antibiotics will then not be effective in treating diseases caused by the bacteria. Examples that many will be familiar with are MRSA (methi-cillin-resistant staphylococcus aureus) and XDR-TB (extensively drug-resistant tuberculosis), while salmonella species also commonly demonstrate antibiotic resistance. The increase in resistance will reduce the antibiotics that can be used. Many antibiotics are also used in human medicine and there is increasing pressure to remove the antibiotics from use by veterinary surgeons. The evidence that resistance appearing in humans is caused by the overuse of antibiotics in animals is limited. However, good antibiotic stewardship would appear to be a sensible approach in order to protect the use of these important medications. This includes using them only when required (not as a panacea for poor animal keeping), dispensing adequate doses, ensuring compliance with treatment plans and testing for resistance where it is suspected.

Another class of medications that are in danger of becoming useless to the veterinary and farming professions are the anthelmintics. These are used to kill worms in the stomach and intestines in order to protect the welfare and production of grazing animals. This is going to be an important function in the future as food production becomes more important as climate change changes the range of parasites and puts pressure on the available land for food production. There are five different types of these anthelmintics available to treat the grazing animal population and the first type of these were discovered (benzimidazoles) in the 1960s and this class of anthelmintics has on many farms ceased to be able to kill the parasites in the ruminants (particularly sheep). Of the remaining four classes, when surveillance (either passive or active) has been carried out, resistant worms have been found for all of them. One of the most recently released classes on the market – amino-acetonitrile derivatives, released onto the European market around 2010 – is already compromised as an effective treatment with resistant worms documented in Europe and New Zealand. This leaves one class of anthelmintics for which there are no known resistant worms, so the temptation is to rely on this medication for treating all animals. But this will run the risk of losing even this final medication. There are major initiatives and discussions in order to minimise the further spread of resistance on farms throughout the world.

One of the future challenges that the veterinary profession faces will be to preserve the utility of these medications, either anthelmintic treatments or antibiotics, from either irresponsible use or overuse. This will be important in protecting human and animal health, as antibiotics are directly useful for human medicine and anthelmintic resistance in gut worms will reduce the ability of farming to feed the human population.

Treating animals (and humans) leaves residues within the tissues of the animals treated. When these animals are used for human consumption then the levels of medications detectable should be below specified levels. These levels are frequently under review with the relevant competent authorities and it may be decided that there is no acceptable upper limit for residues then these medications may be removed from use in animals intended for human consumption. This will pose challenges for the profession as a whole, including replacing the medication with a viable alternative, and educating and enforcing the new medication rules.

This residue issue may well have an impact beyond the food production work carried out by veterinary surgeons. The residues that are left in the carcase have been associated with impacts on the wildlife. Diclofenac, a non-steroidal drug with similar clinical effects to aspirin and ibuprofen, has been shown to kill vultures. This has been seen in the Indian subcontinent and is of concern in Europe where some vulture species are endangered. At a smaller scale, some of the macrocyclic lactone class of wormers can have an impact on the invertebrate population of snails. These are the first interactions that have been identified and take veterinary treatment considerations to a global level.

Some treatment used in veterinary medicine might cause concern for the profession, yet are popular with many members of the public and a minority of the profession. For example, there has been a recent upsurge in the debate over the use of homeopathy and homeopathic remedies. These medications have no detectable ingredient in the prescribed medicine (either a pill or a water dose) and theoretical calculations suggest that no active ingredient would be found in the output of a major homeopathic remedy manufacturer. There have been veterinary advocates that have made considerable noise about having speaking engagements at conferences cancelled and have suggested academic suppression. The use of homeopathic medicine sits uncomfortably with an evidence-based profession. As the veterinary surgeons trained in assessing evidence and the underlying research base look at the issue then the use of treatment modality will reduce. Before this happens, however, there will be robust discussion within the profession. Homeopathy is only one of a number of interventions that are not actively harmful but may delay the animal getting appropriate treatment. Reiki, acupuncture and herbal medicines are probably the next most popular but there are more. There will always be public pressure to offer these treatments but where they sit in a science and evidence-based profession is a matter for self-reflection by the profession.

While animal vaccination is a very useful tool for preventing medicine, it has similar issues to those seen in human vaccination. In certain areas there is a reduction in the number of animals being vaccinated due to a belief that vaccination is associated with an increased risk of other diseases such as cancers and autoimmune disorders. While no intervention is without risk, the benefits of vaccination outweigh any problems and generally – with the exception of a few well-defined problems – the issues are illusory. The role of the veterinary surgeon in the future will be to communicate the science on any issue accurately and well. This is needed to maintain vaccination rates but will become more difficult in the future as the science becomes more complex.

There is always a social good to veterinary practice and working with companion animals is part of this, which is widely accepted. Companion animals have found roles as therapeutic animals in hospices and care homes. While treating these animals is a pleasant aspect to this social responsibility role there are, however, less pleasant parts to this. Many child abusers and some who go on to kill have started with harming animals. There is a link between cruelty to animals and abuse towards children and partners either at the same time or later in life. Working out how to determine whether this is happening and how to deal with it is an area where the profession is actively debating and working with the medical profession to develop best practice guidelines to protect humans and animals.

The overall theme of change within veterinary practice might be a shift to an advisory role from a medicine sales role. The service offered would follow the dentist model and centre on the preventative advice that a veterinary surgeon can offer. The best payment model that will develop around this is still to be determined and will probably be decided at an individual practice level.

BOVINE TUBERCULOSIS IN THE UK

A disease that is currently causing a problem worldwide and will continue to be a problem for the foreseeable future is bovine tuberculosis (bovine TB). This disease has many characteristics that make it more difficult to manage. The difficulties with the control of bovine TB start with the inability to treat it as the antibiotics are expensive, unreliable, have no licence for use in food-producing animals and are ultimately uneconomic to use. These difficulties continue to diagnostic techniques that are relatively crude in comparison to more recently developed diagnostics tests. Bovine TB takes a long time from the point of infection to the clinical signs appearing and this can also complicate detection. The understanding of the risks associated with bovine TB is also unclear and in particular the interaction with other species and with wildlife. Politically there is a great debate about how to manage the disease and this leads to frustration on all sides, with farmers potentially taking matters into their own hands by targeting badgers. Other have viewed this as a way to make money by swapping ear tags in cattle and injecting substances to change the results. The future of this disease may have a massive impact on the future of farming in the UK and wherever it may spread.

In the UK, debate has focused on the control of the disease in wildlife. The European badger is infected with bovine TB and can pass the disease to other badgers, cattle or other species. A current strand of thinking is that the removal (culling/killing) of a large enough number of badgers will reduce the amount of disease in the animal population as a whole and reduce the overall rate of infection. Large-scale experiments looking at the effect of culling have led to ambiguous results and a cost-effective method to kill the badgers that meets criteria that includes the humaneness of the method have proved difficult to find. Research is ongoing to allow the targeting and removal of infected badgers rather than the blanket culling over a large area. Animal rights groups and badger protection organisations all object for a variety of reasons to the mass killing of an iconic British land mammal. Some will accept that the badgers suffer from this disease as well as cattle and other farmed species; as with cattle, treating wildlife is not possible due to the length of time treatment is required for. If it were possible to identify specific diseased individuals, the public acceptance of this approach may increase as removing diseased animals will improve the welfare of the badger population as a whole and protect the cattle population. The current administration in England has planned to roll out a large-scale culling project but the effectiveness and ability to deliver are both in question and badger culling over large areas of England is unlikely.

Protecting the population of cattle would be helped if there were a vaccination available that was acceptable to the international trading partners and animal health regulators. A vaccine is being tested that it is hoped will allow protection of cattle. The vaccine is also designed to allow differentiation between vaccinated and infected cattle. The acceptance of this vaccine will require the data from scientists conducting the field trials and the work of government vets negotiating the complex international politics to get the rules changed to allow the trading of vaccinated animals.

Vaccines for cattle will help but other farmed species are also becoming increasingly infected with the microorganism that causes bovine TB (*mycobacterium bovis*). Currently no controls are in place within the UK for other species and, due to the testing limitations, no country tests all the animals that could become infected. A future direction could be a comprehensive testing programme covering all farmed species including deer, sheep goats, camelids (alpacas, llamas) and pigs. This may be combined with some form of wildlife surveillance. Any programme this comprehensive will require investment and currently this may be difficult unless the economic outlook changes. Most countries are looking to trim budgets and reduce governmental costs. Control of bovine TB has been no exception and this will change the manner of delivery with impacts that are not yet found. The testing was traditionally carried out by the veterinary surgeon who would normally treat the animals on the farm. This task was put out to tender by the government in an efficiency and cost-saving measure. The tender process was won in England by a company that allows the farmer to choose which veterinary surgeon is to carry out the bovine TB testing on the farms. In Scotland and Wales, the veterinary surgeons collaborated to win the tender, so that the farm veterinary surgeons still deliver the bovine TB testing regime. What effect this will have on the bovine TB testing results is very difficult to predict. The professionalism of the veterinary profession will ensure that the testing results are as reliable as it is possible to make them. This change to the bovine TB testing regime was viewed with some trepidation by the profession. Removing bovine TB testing was anticipated to reduce the income of practices if the testing function was taken by another organisation. Some practices will see a potential reduction in income as farmers use another veterinary surgeon to carry out the testing. The final impact of the changes will become apparent over the coming years.

Cattle controls are going to remain key to the control of bovine TB in the future. Animals will be checked on a regular basis, carried out by the veterinary surgeons belonging to the organisations that won the tenders. The frequency of testing may change and become more frequent. Movement may only be permitted after testing of the individual and all animals may be tested after the movement has been completed. Some countries already carry out this but this may be taken across all the UK. The results of these tests are currently confidential but allowing purchasers of cattle to know the bovine TB pattern on the farm where any cattle have originated from will allow an assessment of the risk attached to the purchase. This change may encourage the change to a risk-based trading approach with an assessment of disease risk and this can be an approach that can be transferred to other diseases. Interactions with wildlife can introduce infection within herds. Veterinary surgeons are able to give advice to control these interactions and as experience as a profession is gained by both veterinary surgeons and farmers, this advice will improve and have a better effect on the overall disease picture.

The ultimate aim of these changes is to eradicate bovine TB and in the UK the chief veterinary officers of England has stated that they would like to see the country achieving Officially Bovine Tuberculosis Free (OTF) status by 2038. There are areas of the UK where the trend is suggestive that this aim will be achieved. The current state of play with this disease is that the pattern for England as a whole is stable. Some areas have a downward trend and others are getting worse. Wales as a whole has a downward trend and hopefully this will continue over the next years. Scotland has achieved OTF status and this is something that should be protected.

Bovine TB control has many lessons that may be learnt by the profession in the future, from cost-sharing and new ways to manage wildlife interactions to risk-based trading. It is to be hoped that all these lessons will result in a disease-free herd.

SUMMARY

The prediction of the future is almost guaranteed to be wrong and the further ahead we look, the less likely it is that a specific prediction will be right. Some things can be guessed at with some confidence, such as increasing numbers and changes in the gender ratio of the profession. Other things are inevitable in general but impossible to determine in detail. It is inevitable that we will see novel diseases but when and of what type is impossible to determine. All of the points discussed here have that problem and if another Veterinary Surgeon was asked to compile a similar list it could look completely different.

14
SUMMARY

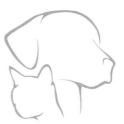

Working as a veterinary surgeon is an incredibly rewarding position to find yourself in. I have been one for 15 years now and every day I have gone to work looking forward to the challenge ahead. . . well, at least most days I look forward to the job. It's only recently that veterinary surgeons have felt the confidence to start a realistic conversation about the pressures and issues that we as a profession face. One of the thought processes that made me write this book was the chance to try and let a prospective veterinary student or their relatives get some ink- ling of the true nature of the career. This is a personal view but is based on 15 years of involvement in the profession and I have worked in almost all aspects of veterinary medicine from small animal corporate practice to research and teach- ing in farm animal medicine. I have been involved in abattoir work and inspected factories and consignments to allow export of fish from the Atlantic Ocean to Russia. Veterinary politics has also become part of my professional career, working with governments and the profession as a whole to develop responses to issues that are of concern. So I hope that I have a reasonable background to allow me to give an overview of the profession and present a view that is neither too opti- mistic nor too pessimistic. Since I have qualified, too many of my classmates and colleagues have been lost to the profession through deciding that they no longer wish to work and, tragically, through suicide. The major contributor to this is the pressure of the job but another factor, in my view, is a mismatch between what the prospective veterinary surgeon applying to the course expects and the actual course or career. This book is an attempt to address this gap that I see with stu- dents. I hope that it allows you as a prospective veterinary student or as a person supporting a prospective student to start thinking about the issues a student and qualified veterinary surgeon faces and make a rational and justified decision based on your reading of this book and other information that you may come across.

Veterinary surgeons are primarily thought of as curing animals and this would be the stereotypically James Herriot image and the image that many members of the public have when they picture a veterinary surgeon. The veterinary surgeon in a consulting room will remain an important part of the profession and the diagnostic skills that are taught and have been part of veterinary medicine for years will remain vital. Stethoscopes will be used to listen to chests and abdomens to determine the functioning of the internal organs. Blood samples will be analysed for an increasing numbers of things. There will always be interventions and these will change as research into the treatment of diseases reaches the frontline of veterinary practice. The type of animal will change as exotic pets fall in and out of fashion with the public. Advice to owners will change in response to new research ideas or legislation, from treatment advice to advice that is more preventative in nature. This will require an increasingly sophisticated understanding of the epidemiological concepts associated with disease and treatment. Evidence-based medicine will become a more central concept, with clinical governance and self-critical assessment of personal practices becoming more common at a practice level. This self-critical assessment should allow effective practices to be identified not only by research but by looking at what occurs in the practice or on the farms that the veterinary surgeons work on. This may be a painful experience as treasured remedies or techniques may be shown to be ineffective (or dangerous) and have to be discarded. But the profession will be better for it.

The day-to-day profession has many pressures. Clients can also be extremely critical and put an unreasonable amount of pressure on the veterinary surgeon. There will be cases where whatever is done the animal will die (or treatment will fail) through no fault of the treating veterinary surgeon and the owners will look to blame someone. This reaction may be a natural reaction to the grief of losing an animal, an expression of other issues in the owner's life such as overwhelming debt or it may be malicious. Whatever the reason for the desire to hit out, the situation places a great deal of stress on the veterinary surgeon and this can lead to depression and other forms of mental illness. Coping mechanisms that are used can include sports, family and friends and other outside and constructive interests. If these are not there or are not sufficient to help cope then more destructive coping mechanisms may be used such as excessive drinking, use of narcotic substances and – in some very tragic cases – suicide. The suicide rate of the profession is higher than we would like, and a number of organisations are working to change this.

There are other ways to work with animals after getting your veterinary degree. Although these have been looked on as second-class jobs by some in the veterinary profession, this will change as the increase in number of qualifying students increases. The range of animal specific careers that veterinary qualified graduates can apply to is huge and important. If you choose to go to a veterinary course then the options include research into almost any biological area, protecting the food that we eat or specialising in one area of veterinary medicine. Some will leave the profession and do something else instead. There are veterinary surgeons that have gone on to be religious minsters, work in finance and probably many more.

The profession is a difficult one but it adds a massive amount to the world as a whole. Companion animal practice enriches the social life of many people by caring for their pets. The care of companion animals is a social good in helping all of its members to live a good life. Food production also requires the input of veterinary surgeons to protect the welfare of the animals from the farm all the way to the abattoir. This addition to the human food chain can mean the survival of people. Veterinary surgeons working in conservation and with wildlife can contribute to the survival of species and the environment that they live in. The local human population can also be supported by veterinary surgeons in allowing animals in these areas to coexist successfully.

All of these careers and tasks carried out by veterinary surgeons – whether they are in a clinical setting in the UK or USA, whether they are on a farm or in companion animal clinics, working in research or the myriad other areas – will have ethical implications. The underpinnings of an individual's worldview can be different from a religious view or a deep consideration of the philosophical thinking or just simply considering the animal as a sentient being worthy of respect and good treatment. The application of these principles by veterinary surgeons tends to result in animals being treated with skill and compassion; this minimises the suffering that the animal experiences. 'Minimises' can be a difficult concept in some cases and particularly in research there are determined efforts to reduce the use of animals. In companion and farm animals the responsibility is increasingly being placed on owners but the veterinary surgeon has to guide the owner to a decision that is best for all concerned.

This is closely allied to the welfare of the animals and the concept of a good life. What makes an animal's existence a 'good life' is open to some debate when it comes to definitions, even though it seems obvious when an animal is observed that it has a good life. The welfare of animals is of most concern in food producing species as there is a good deal of attention associated with these species. There are numerous guides and codes to help keepers and veterinary surgeons work together to improve the welfare of the animals. This area is probably the important part of the veterinary surgeon's role, as many oaths that they swear on entering the profession make reference to the welfare of the animals that are under their care. What is good welfare will change in response to the new thinking about how society keeps animals. This may be a change in the attitude to companion animals such as dogs that are bred with characteristics that may cause health issues, the use of exotic animals as novel pets or new ways of farming animals for food or fibre. Ensuring that this is carried out in a way that does not compromise the welfare of animals will be at the heart of the veterinary surgeon's role whether this is in dealing with individual animals or working with governments and non-governmental organisations to promote good welfare. This will interact with their role in the political life where veterinary surgeons work with government to deal with the issues and try to manage the competing pressures on society. It will require the continued skill of veterinary surgeons with many types of expertise to ensure that the improvements the profession wants to see are continued without damaging the independence of the profession.

The media will continue to have an interest in the veterinary profession because of our work with animals, which can be extremely telegenic and of great public interest and our importance in protecting the safety and quality of the food that societies eat. Our position as a profession in commenting on this debate relies on us being generally perceived as honest and fair in our dealings and free of underlying motives such as financial gain.

We work as part of a team as no part of caring for animals is carried out in isolation. Alternatively there might be a surgical team with overlapping and complementary skills working to carry out a complex surgical intervention or it might be a team based on farm working to optimise different parts of the business and there are many other potential examples. The veterinary surgeon has to be able to work in the team or provide leadership as required by the situation. Leadership generally requires a personal style and can be demonstrated in many ways but personal integrity, honesty and respect for others are core to leadership. Within the veterinary practices there are many other professionals from cattle foot trimmers, equine dentists and obviously nurses, and using their skills in the team will allow the best intervention to be developed for the animals concerned.

Veterinary surgeons work in a complex social, political and scientific environment and many will group together to discuss matters of mutual interest and these can be general in membership and interest or for a specialist group. This allows the best consensus answer to many questions. Others will award qualifications or certify institutions as being of sufficient standard whether these are veterinary practices or universities that train veterinary surgeons.

That is the overview of the profession that I have tried to give in this book. The profession is a rewarding one but it has difficulties and challenges. This level of challenge along with the massive amount of science and interpersonal skills means that the profession needs high quality candidates to enter the profession. Academic qualifications are key to this but gradually there is a feeling that these are insufficient. It is unlikely that even if there are a large number of vet schools anything less than a full suite of top grades is going to be sufficient. Alongside this, experience of the profession in some manner is going to be required but in the future more rigorous selection procedures may be used to identify the correct students. The course will still have the recognisable core subjects such as anatomy, biochemistry and animal husbandry. Whether all students will be exposed to the details from all species or whether they will specialise early into specific species groups will be one possibility that may occur. How the subjects are taught will vary from university to university but will be informed by new educational techniques even though the evidence for these can be difficult to determine.

How all of veterinary medicine is paid for is always a difficult question. Clients with animals that die may well feel that they should not have to pay and many others when presented with the costs will feel that they are too high. The value of the services that veterinary surgeons provide must be communicated – especially when compared to the medical profession. What services we are selling will change, with more veterinary surgeons moving to charging for advice only. The way owners budget for this will change and insurance models may change to get more owners to invest in this protection. Practices may also try to increase the preventative advice given to companion animal owners and charge monthly subscription fees to visit the practice. Other ways of paying may be developed but they will have to deliver a benefit and this philosophy extends all the way to government-sponsored programmes that are expected to demonstrate a benefit of some kind but most commonly economic.

When you enter veterinary school there will be some financial issues to contend with. The level of fees is likely to increase unless capped by the government in a particular country. I can't see this happening in the UK and this appears to be the only country where the discussion is happening. Financing this can come from financial companies, government loan organisations, sponsorship and other more individual sources. The majority of these will require the repayment of the capital borrowed and the salary earned will have to be used to repay the borrowing. Whether this is going to be possible is increasingly unlikely for some, particularly those that are paying the full fees on a second course. The careers that you will be entering are much wider than the veterinary surgeon examining a cat or dog or performing a caesarean section on a cow. These new opportunities are just as valuable to the public in protecting the health of people. In fact the veterinary medicine course is able to take the holder into many areas of human endeavour as it is at the very least a high-quality science qualification.

I hope this book allows you to make an informed choice about whether to join the profession. The future of the profession is in the hands of those that join it over the coming years. Future vets will have to have many of the skills that previous generations have worked hard to develop and a whole suite that the future veterinary surgeons will develop through hard work, critical self-reflection and research. The future challenges of the profession will need talented and dedicated people who are robust enough to deal with the changing circumstances that personal lives and the global changes will throw at them. The reward will be a challenging and rewarding career that brings respect from all parts of societies and now it comes with the title of 'doctor' when you qualify!

APPENDIX 1 –
RUMA GUIDELINES

The Responsible Use of Medicines in Agriculture Alliance (RUMA) was established in November 1997 to promote the highest standards of food safety, animal health and animal welfare in British livestock farming.

A unique initiative involving organisations representing every stage of the food chain, RUMA aims to produce a coordinated and integrated approach to best practice in the use of medicines.

RESPONSIBLE USE OF ANTIMICROBIALS IN DAIRY AND BEEF CATTLE PRODUCTION

This appendix summarises the farmer's responsibility as part of the RUMA guidelines for the responsible use of antimicrobials in dairy and beef cattle production.

Antimicrobials have made a major contribution to cattle health and welfare. They are vital medicines for the treatment of bacterial infections in cattle.

The emergence of antimicrobial resistance as a serious problem in human medicine has prompted concerns about the potential for crossover of resistant bacteria from livestock to the human population and the associated possibility of this impacting on the effectiveness of medical antimicrobial treatments.

RUMA is a coalition of organisations including agricultural, veterinary, pharmaceutical, retail and consumer interests.

It has been set up to review the use of medicines in livestock and to establish practical strategies to reduce the need to use antimicrobials.

To meet this end, RUMA has produced a comprehensive set of guidelines for the responsible use of antimicrobials in livestock production. These give advice on all aspects from application and responsibilities of farmers and veterinary surgeons, to strategies for reducing the need for usage.

This appendix summarises responsibilities of dairy and beef farmers. Similar guidelines form part of farm assurance schemes.

The guidelines

- There is a joint responsibility between the veterinary surgeon and the farmer to ensure that antimicrobials are used correctly and for the right reason. Ultimately, it is the farmer who is responsible for ensuring that animal medicines are used in a safe, responsible and effective way on the farm.

- Dairy and beef farmers are committed to ensuring the safety of food they produce for consumers.

- Farmers have a responsibility to safeguard the health of the animals on their farm.

- Therapeutic antimicrobial products should be regarded as complementing good management and farm hygiene. Herd health plans should be drawn up and include routine preventative treatments (e.g., routine foot care, mastitis, vaccination and worming).

- Treatment should be initiated with a medicine that is subject to veterinary prescription only with formal veterinary approval. Accurate information, including other medicines being administered, should be given to the veterinary surgeon to allow correct diagnosis and appropriate medication and dosage. Clear instructions must be left on the farm and made available to all staff responsible.

- The full course of treatment at the correct dosage should always be administered.

- The appropriate withdrawal period prior to slaughter, or for the sale of milk for human consumption, must be ensured. Information on the required withdrawal period can be found on the medicine labels.

- An animal medicines record book together with copies of relevant regulations and Codes of Practice must be kept on the farm.

- Accurately record the identity of the treated animals, the batch number, amount and expiry date of the medicine used, plus the required withdrawal period and the time and date the medication was completed for any specific animal. Appropriate information should be kept on file of medicines used (e.g., product data sheets, package inserts or safety data sheets). Records must be kept for a period of five years after the treatment has ended even if the animal has been slaughtered.

- Medicines must be stored according to the manufacturers' instructions. Unused or unwanted medicines must be disposed of according to manufacturers' instructions or returned to the veterinary surgeon or supplier for safe disposal.

- Any suspected adverse reactions in either the animals undergoing treatment or the staff treating them, should be reported to the Veterinary Medicines Directorate (VMD).

- Adverse reaction forms can be found on the VMD's website, www.vmd.gov.uk. A report can be submitted by the farmer or the attending veterinary surgeon. Keep a note in the medicines book or a copy of the VMD adverse reaction report if available.

- Cooperate with Farm Assurance Schemes that monitor medication and withdrawal compliance. However, such schemes should not constrain the farmer from preventing the suffering of animals.

- Work with the veterinary surgeon in monitoring the potency of antimicrobial use.

The guidelines assume that the antimicrobial substances available are officially authorised for the purpose for which they are used and that they are lawfully obtained.

The use of animal medicines carries with it responsibilities. Under UK legislation, all antimicrobials are licensed for specific species and uses. A product will not be authorised unless very astringent requirements are met. The use of therapeutic antimicrobials is under the direct responsibility of veterinary surgeons. Farmers, however, have a very considerable role to play in ensuring that the directions of the veterinary surgeon are properly carried out and also in developing and applying disease control measures which minimise the need for antimicrobial use.

RUMA Responsible Use Guidelines are also available for all the main livestock species at RUMA's website, www.ruma.org.uk.

APPENDIX 2 – BSAVA STATEMENT

TABLE A1

Title	*Complementary and alternative therapies*
Statement	The British Small Animal Veterinary Association (BSAVA) recognises that owners may seek alternative and complementary therapies for their animals for a wide range of reasons, however in the interests of animal welfare:
	The BSAVA recommends that owners consider the evidence for a particular treatment and the qualifications and experience of the practitioner before embarking on any complementary or alternative therapy for their pet.
	The BSAVA strongly recommends that treatment of animals is only undertaken after appropriate assessment and diagnosis by a veterinary surgeon.
	The BSAVA strongly recommends that whenever possible treatment decisions are based on sound scientific evidence to support the safety and efficacy of the therapy.
	The BSAVA strongly recommends that owners should seek advice from their veterinary surgeon before using any form of complementary or alternative therapy in their animals.
Background information	**Legal situation**
	The diagnosis of diseases in and injuries to animals (including tests performed on animals for diagnostic purposes), as well as giving advice based upon such diagnosis, and the medical or surgical treatment of animals, are considered to be acts of 'veterinary surgery' as defined by Section 19 of the Veterinary Surgeons Act 1966. Subject to a small number of exceptions diagnosis and treatment of animals may only be carried out by registered members of the Royal College of Veterinary Surgeons (RCVS).

TABLE A1 continued

Title	Complementary and alternative therapies

Background information	The Animal Welfare Act 2006 imposes a duty on the owner of or other person in charge of an animal to ensure that its welfare needs are met. This includes the need to be protected from pain, suffering, injury and disease.

Veterinary medicinal products are defined as any *substance or combination of substances presented as having properties for treating or preventing disease in animals; or any substance or combination of substances that may be used in, or administered to, animals with a view either to restoring, correcting or modifying physiological functions by exerting a pharmacological, immunological or metabolic action, or to making a medical diagnosis.* In the UK these products are subject to control on the manufacture, authorisation, marketing, distribution and post-authorisation surveillance as detailed in the Veterinary Medicines Regulations.

What is meant by complementary and alternative medicine

Complementary and alternative therapies are a diverse group of practices and products not considered part of conventional (mainstream) medicine. Although 'complementary and alternative' is often used as a single category, it can be useful to make a distinction between the two different ways of using these treatments.

Complementary therapies are used together with conventional medicine while alternative therapies are used instead of conventional medicine, although they are sometimes used at the same time as, but not in deliberate concert with, conventional medicine. 'Integrative medicine' is a term used to refer to treatments that combine conventional medicine with those complementary therapies for which there is reasonable evidence of safety and effectiveness.

Safety and efficacy

Health claims for many complementary and alternative therapies are far in excess of the available scientific data, and sometimes in frank contradiction to scientific evidence.

In making decisions about the use of complementary and alternative therapies, it is important to consider their safety and efficacy. Many people assume that all complementary and alternative therapies are natural and therefore safe, but this is not always the case. All therapies may produce unwanted side-effects or may interact with other therapies. In the case of alternative therapies it is also important to consider the welfare implications of withholding conventional treatments.

Title	*Complementary and alternative therapies*
Background information	There is a great deal of variation in both the degree to which various complementary and alternative therapies have been scientifically tested, and to which such testing has provided evidence supporting their efficacy. Establishing the efficacy of a therapy is not always straightforward; many conditions may fluctuate over time or resolve on their own.

Within any one branch of complementary medicine, for example, herbal remedies or physiotherapy, there may be products or procedures with reasonable evidence of efficacy and safety for certain conditions, but others for which the evidence is poor or indicates that the product or procedure is ineffective.

Assessing the evidence

Some people, including owners, therapists and veterinary surgeons, may perceive that the therapies work as a result of belief in the therapy (placebo effect), anecdotal evidence (extrapolation from hearsay or personal experience of a single or small number of cases) or errors in inference (cognitive bias).

There are three factors strongly associated with whether or not any one medical treatment is likely to be efficacious:

1. A rational scientific basis

Modern medicine works, and it works because it is founded on a scientific base. Although not all treatments used in conventional medicine have a strong evidence base in the sense of rigorous clinical trials showing their efficacy they do have a rational scientific/pathophysiological basis for their use.

2. Degree of certainty

The effects of some treatments are so clear cut that further testing is not required. It has famously been pointed out that rigorous clinical trials are not needed to prove that parachutes reduce morbidity and mortality among people falling from aeroplanes. Similarly, one does not need rigorous trials to show that intravenous anaesthetics cause a rapid, profound loss of consciousness suitable for carrying out surgery. However, the effects of many treatments are much less certain; for example, they are less closely associated in time with their effect, or the effect caused is much less dramatic, smaller and/or more variable in magnitude and/or time of onset. In such circumstances, given the variable time courses of many diseases, it can be remarkably difficult to determine whether a given treatment is actually efficacious or not.

Title	*Complementary and alternative therapies*

Background information	**3. Evidence**

When there is anything less than absolute certainty about the efficacy of a treatment, then evidence is important in deciding whether a treatment is safe and efficacious. However, history has also shown that evidence – both in the form of clinical experience and individual clinical research results – can be misleading. The process of evidence-based (veterinary) medicine exists to improve our confidence by formally and systematically searching for all of the relevant evidence and formally and systematically grading the quality and reliability of that evidence.

Choosing a practitioner

Regulation exists to protect patient safety: it does not by itself mean that there is scientific evidence that a treatment is effective.

Currently, practitioners of two complementary and alternative medicines are regulated in the same way as practitioners of conventional medicine. They are osteopathy and chiropractic. This regulation is called statutory professional regulation.

If you want to use a complementary and alternative medicine where practitioners are not regulated by professional statutory regulation, you should make use of professional bodies or voluntary registers, where they exist, to help you find a practitioner.

You may want to check what arrangements there are for complaining about a practitioner. For example, does the association or register accept complaints, and what action will they take if you have concerns about your treatment?

Related statements	Referral to para-professionals
Websites	Further information about the Veterinary Surgeon's Act and complementary therapy can be found on the RCVS website
	Animal Welfare Act
	Further information on the regulations relating to veterinary medicines can be found on the website of the Veterinary Medicines Directorate (VMD)
Provenance	Scientific Committee 2013
	BSAVA Council November 2013

This document is also available on www.bsava.com/Resources/Positionstatements (accessed on 22 May 2015).

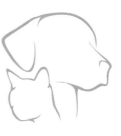

USEFUL SOURCES OF INFORMATION

APPLYING TO UNIVERSITY

The websites below will give more information about the application process and its various parts.

www.ucas.com
www.aavmc.org/Students-Applicants-and-Advisors/Veterinary-Medical-College-Application-Service.aspx
www.admissionstestingservice.org/for-test-takers/bmat/about-bmat

VET SCHOOL WEBSITES

Links to the various vet schools that you can apply to.

UK

www.bristol.ac.uk/vetscience
www.vet.cam.ac.uk
www.ed.ac.uk/schools-departments/vet/services
www.gla.ac.uk/schools/vet
www.liv.ac.uk/veterinary-science
www.nottingham.ac.uk/vet/index.aspx
www.rvc.ac.uk
www.surrey.ac.uk/vet

Ireland

www.ucd.ie/vetmed

New Zealand

www.massey.ac.nz/massey/learning/colleges/college-of-sciences/students/
vetschool/vetschool_home.cfm

Australia

www.uq.edu.au/vetschool
http://sydney.edu.au/vetscience
www.murdoch.edu.au/School-of-Veterinary-and-Life-Sciences
www.adelaide.edu.au/vetsci
www.csu.edu.au/courses/vet-science-biology
www-public.jcu.edu.au/courses/health/vet/index.htm
http://fvas.unimelb.edu.au

USA

There are many universities that offer veterinary courses, the link below gives a list.

www.avma.org/professionaldevelopment/education/accreditation/colleges/
pages/colleges-accredited.aspx

REGULATORY BODIES

These organisations will licence the veterinary surgeons in their country.

www.rcvs.org.uk/home
www.avbc.asn.au
www.vetcouncil.org.nz
www.nbvme.org

PROFESSIONAL BODIES

These organisations will represent the veterinary profession to the government and public.

www.avma.org/Pages/home.aspx
www.bva.co.uk
www.ava.com.au
www.nzva.org.nz
www.canadianveterinarians.net

ALLIED ORGANISATIONS

The organisations that work alongside veterinary surgeons and will give more information about what they do.

www.vetfutures.org.uk
www.bvna.org.uk
www.nacft.co.uk/wp
www.acpat.org
www.navp.co.uk
www.baedt.com
www.apbc.org.uk

WEBSITES WITH CLINICAL INFORMATION

To find out more about diseases of animals, these websites are useful.

www.nadis.org.uk
www.merckmanuals.com/vet
http://en.wikivet.net/Veterinary_Education_Online

SPECIALIST VETERINARY ORGANISATIONS

To learn more about what different specialisms in veterinary medicine do these websites will give more information.

www.agv.org.uk
www.avsukireland.co.uk
www.bcva.eu/bcva
www.beva.org.uk/home
www.bsava.com
www.bvba.org.uk
www.bvha.org.uk
www.bvpa.org.uk
www.bvzs.org
www.fishvetsociety.org.uk
www.goatvetsoc.co.uk
www.lava.uk.net
www.pigvetsoc.org.uk
www.army.mod.uk/medical-services/veterinary.aspx
www.sheepvetsoc.org.uk
www.spvs.org.uk
www.vetdeersociety.com
www.vpha.org.uk

A website that details the equivalent organisations in the USA.

www.avma.org/About/AlliedOrganizations/Pages/Allied-Veterinary-Medical-Associations.aspx

GOVERNMENT ORGANISATIONS

These are organisations that apply rules to animals and conduct surveillance of diseases in their countries. They also employ veterinary surgeons.

www.gov.uk/government/organisations/department-for-environment-food-rural-affairs
www.gov.uk/government/organisations/animal-and-plant-health-agency
www.mpi.govt.nz
www.australia.gov.au/topics/business-and-industry/primary-industry
www.usda.gov/wps/portal/usda/usdahome

DEVELOPMENT ORGANISATIONS

These are organisations that are working to improve animal health and welfare throughout the world.

www.galvmed.org
www.rvc.ac.uk/Global/KenyaDroughtAppeal/VetAidKenya.cfm
www.vsfe.org
www.veterinairessansfrontieres.be
www.vetswithoutborders.ca
www.missionrabies.com
wvs.org.uk
spana.org
www.thebrooke.org
www.gambiahorseanddonkey.org.uk
www.sendacow.org

INDEX

CPD *see* continuous professional
    development
CVS 92

Dangerous Dog Act (1991) 51
day one competencies 21
Defra *see* Department for Environment
    Farming and Rural Affairs
Department for Environment Farming and
    Rural Affairs (Defra) 57, 79
dermatology 20
Descartes, René 148
developing countries 177
    animal-based organisations 182–4
    charitable projects 181–2
    definition and understanding of
        working in 177–9
    motivations for getting involved in 180
    new and emerging diseases 179–80
    personal health and safety 180–1
    training local farmers 178
    and zoonotic disease 179
diagnostic tests 37, 39–40
    costs 123
    culture/sensitivity on swabs/samples 38
    faecal samples 37
    sensitivity/specificity 39
    skin scrapes 38
    snout 39
    spin 39
    urine samples 37
disciplinary matters 74–5
DNA 63
Doctorate in Veterinary Medicine (DVM)
    71
dogs 30, 32, 33, 38, 46, 48, 49, 51, 55, 57,
    59, 60, 61, 65–6, 67, 80, 88, 91,
    108, 109, 130, 136–7, 139, 155–6,
    159, 179
Doherty, Peter Charles 173–4
Domestic Abuse Veterinary Initiative 152
Donkey Sanctuary 108, 182
Dublin University 71, 115
DVM *see* Doctorate in Veterinary Medicine

EAEVE *see* European Association of
    Establishments for Veterinary
    Education
ear-cropping 157
EAVE 21
Ebola 180
economics 112
    charity veterinary medicine 128–30
    cost benefit at national level 130
    cost benefit for production animals 130
    cost of living at university 116
    cost of studying 113–16, 205–6
    cost of treating animals 122–6, 205
    cost-sharing 131
    expected salary 117–22
    paying for training 117
    polluter pays concept 131
    running a practice 126–8
    summary of issues 131–2
    who should pay 131
Edinburgh University 71, 114, 167
EIA (equine infectious anaemia) 88
EMS *see* extra mural studies
environmental safety 82–3
epidemiology 19
equine dentist 57–8
equine physiotherapist 60
equine racing industry 135–6
equine veterinary surgeon 57, 58, 96, 118
ethics 19
    discussion concerning 139–40
    frameworks 133–4
    in medicine 143
    open and honest 134
    procedures 139
    and religion 141–3
    research 138–9
    societal interaction 140
    use of animals 134–7
    wildlife interaction 140–1
European Association of Establishments
    for Veterinary Education (EAEVE)
    72, 77
European directives 21